CAREGIVING FOR ALZHEIMER'S DISEASE: A PERSONAL JOURNEY

by
William L. Harris

Acknowledgments

I want to thank Anne Harris for editing and Heather Pendley of Pendley's Pro Editing & Indexing for whipping this book into shape and indexing this book. I would also like to thank my wife, Marilyn, for her encouragement and support. I also need to thank all of the people who participated in Alzheimer's support groups who provided invaluable insight, wisdom and compassion for each other.

Dedicated to Nora R. Harris
February 1953 – October 2017
diagnosed with early onset Alzheimer's disease July 2009

CONTENTS

TABLE OF FIGURES

FOREWORD

Who I Am

I am William Harris, 79 years old. I graduated from the University of Oregon with bachelor's (1964) and master's (1965) degrees in political science, but through a circuitous route, wound up in information technology in the financial industry. I retired from Wells Fargo Bank on December 31, 2016, after working there 25 years. I planned to retire at 67, but my wife, Nora, was diagnosed with early onset Alzheimer's disease. Knowing that I would have to pay out-of-pocket for her care, I worked an additional eight years to have the necessary resources.

Many do not have this capability to work longer or have access to sufficient resources. Knowing what she wanted, as per her advance directive, and the usual progression of the disease, I hoped that working until 75 would be sufficient.

I started and facilitated four Alzheimer's disease support groups for caregivers with the cooperation of the Southern Oregon Alzheimer's Association. There are two groups in Medford; one at the senior center and the other at Rogue Valley Manor. There are also two in Ashland.

Who I Am Not

I am not a doctor and do not have formal medical training. Nora was diagnosed at the University of California San Francisco Medical School (UCSF). I have been deeply involved with the medical care of my family and spouse and this has provided me with more insight into the workings of dementia and the medical profession.

I am not a lawyer. However, I have been involved in several legal battles over advance directives and retirement benefits. I have also worked with two different attorneys (one in California, the other in Oregon) in creating the *Harris Family Trust*, our advance directives, and other legal documents. I have also had legal representation in several court sessions. This has provided me with unique insight into the legal profession and its approach to cases involving the care of patients with dementia.

I am not a trained social worker. I have been in therapy for years, developing an understanding of why I feel and act the way I do. Therapy is beneficial when going through very difficult personal issues. I have also developed coping skills and learned how to practice self-care with the help of therapy.

Focus on the Caregiver

Most of the text and examples are focused on the caregiver (and the care receiver, where appropriate.) I hope this book provides a better understanding of the disease and the issues involved with caregiving. We need to also understand the progression of the disease and its effect on behavior. As caregivers, there are many things to think about, understand, and do. In this book, I concentrate on what will confront the caregiver from diagnosis through placement and passing.

The majority of references are internet-based. One can "cut and paste" the URL into the browser to access the site (on digital media) or type the URL into the browser. The remainder of the material is self-taught content—learned by experience—and suggestions on ways to come through this process somewhat whole and vital.

One last thing—I have taught a class, Caregiving for Alzheimer's Disease: A Personal Journey, at Olli (Osher Lifelong Learning Institute) at Southern Oregon University for several years now. I will be teaching this class at SOU in the fall of 2021, and at Olli at George Mason University, Fairfax, Virginia.
We will look at the process chronologically as much as possible.

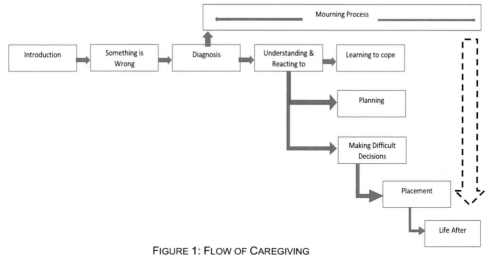

FIGURE 1: FLOW OF CAREGIVING

CHAPTER 1: WHAT CAREGIVERS NEED TO KNOW

A caregiver[1] is a person responsible for the direct care, protection, and supervision of children in childcare or someone who tends to the needs of the elderly or disabled. It is generally one who gives assistance to a person who is no longer able to perform the critical tasks of personal or household care necessary for everyday survival.

Caregivers are governed by federal and state laws, which vary by state, and regulate eligibility and standards of conduct, including areas regarding abuse or neglect of a client or misappropriation of a client's property. A Nevada statute defining a designated primary caregiver (NRS 453A.080) says a "designated primary caregiver" significant responsibility for managing the well-being of a person diagnosed with a chronic or debilitating medical condition, and is designated as such in the manner required pursuant to NRS 453A.250."

The reason for this example is to show that caregiving is a formal activity regulated by the state. You, as a caregiver, are also subject to the same regulations and restrictions. State representatives (ombudsman) can come into your home to review and determine that regulations, restrictions, and general care guidelines are being followed. In other words, they make sure there is no elder abuse.

Effects on Caregivers

I have referenced Maslow's hierarchy of needs to point out some lessons learned from experience and facilitate caregiver support groups. As the disease progresses, the caregiver's needs move down the pyramid toward safety and physiological needs. The demands of caregiving increase over time and will leave little or no time for yourself:

- Your social life shrinks to where you do not invite people over, and go out less
- Guilt and isolation attack your self-esteem; you have less time for your activities, hobbies, and interests
- Intimacy becomes less and less frequent; celibacy may set in; conversation disappears
- Safety becomes a major focus for the loved one; the concern for wandering and/or leaving them alone becomes dominant
- Responsible for meeting the physiological needs of the loved one (meals, personal hygiene, bathing, incontinence, dressing, etc.) may result in neglecting your own physiological needs (i.e., sleep)

---

1 https://definitions.uslegal.com/c/caregiver

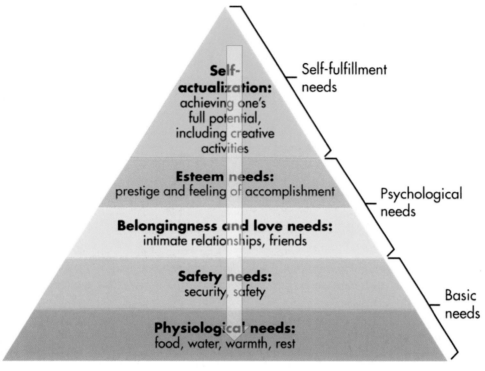

FIGURE 2: MASLOW'S HIERARCHY OF NEEDS[2]

Areas of the Brain[3]

People with dementia have different symptoms depending on the type and stage of their particular dementia and which part of the brain is affected by the disease process. Symptoms may change over time to involve different areas of the brain.

---

2 https://simplypsychology.org/maslow.html
3 https://memory.ucsf.edu/dementia-overview

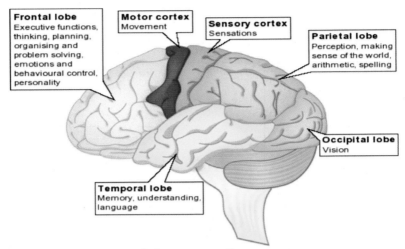

FIGURE 3: AREAS OF THE BRAIN

Different types of dementia tend to target particular parts of the brain. For example, the part of the brain that is important for the formation of new memories is usually affected early on in Alzheimer's disease, which is why short-term memory loss is often one of the first symptoms of the disease.

Other symptoms of dementia often include personality changes, difficulty communicating, planning and organizing, navigation, and psychiatric symptoms such as depression, anxiety, delusions, and hallucinations.

Behavior Areas of the Brain[4]

Behavior and personality often change with dementia; people act in ways that are very different from their "old self," and coping with these changes can be hard for family and friends. With dementia, behavior changes are usually because the person is losing neurons (cells) in parts of their brain. The changes you see often depend on which part of the brain is losing cells.

For example, the frontal lobes are right behind the eyes, which controls our ability to focus, pay attention, be motivated, and other aspects of personality. Therefore, when cells in the

---

4 https://memory.ucsf.edu/behavior-personality-changes

frontal lobes of the brain are lost, people are less able to plan and stay focused. They are less motivated and become more passive. The frontal lobes also control our impulses. Someone with frontal lobe deficits may act rudely or insensitively.

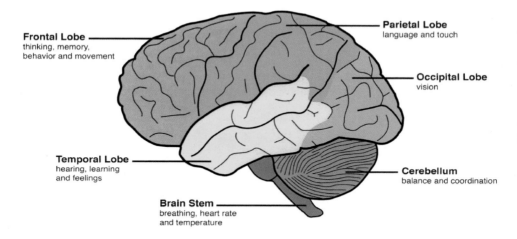

FIGURE 4: BEHAVIOR AREAS OF THE BRAIN

Dementia also alters how a person responds to their environment. A person with Alzheimer's disease may be forgetful and become angry and frustrated because they have trouble following conversations. Noise, conversation, crowds, and activity may be overstimulating and too difficult to process or understand. Also, many people with dementia rely on others for emotional cues. For example, if you are anxious and worried, people with dementia may mirror your emotions and become anxious and worried.

Dynamics of Disease

Mild cognitive impairment (MCI)[5] causes cognitive changes that are serious enough to be noticed by the individuals experiencing them or to other people, but the changes are not severe enough to interfere with daily life or independent function. People with MCI, especially MCI involving memory problems, are more likely to develop Alzheimer's disease or other dementias than people without MCI. However, MCI does not always lead to dementia.

---

5 https://www.alz.org/dementia/mild-cognitive-impairment-mci.asp

In some individuals, MCI remains stable or reverts to normal cognition. In other cases, such as when a medication causes cognitive impairment, MCI is mistakenly diagnosed. That's why it's important that people experiencing cognitive impairment seek help as soon as possible for diagnosis and possible treatment.

Experts classify MCI based on the thinking skills affected:

- MCI that primarily affects memory is known as "amnestic" MCI; a person may start to forget important information that he or she would previously have recalled easily, such as appointments, conversations or recent events

- MCI that affects thinking skills other than memory is known as "non-amnestic" MCI; thinking skills that may be affected include the ability to make sound decisions, judge the time or the sequence of steps needed to complete a complex task, or to perceive things visually

Alzheimer's disease[6] is currently ranked as the sixth leading cause of death in the United States, but recent estimates indicate that the disorder may rank third, just behind heart disease and cancer, as a cause of death for older people. Alzheimer's is the most common cause of dementia among older adults; affecting approximately 5 million people. Dementia is the loss of cognitive functioning—thinking, remembering, and reasoning—and behavioral abilities to such an extent that it interferes with a person's daily life and activities. Dementia ranges in severity from the mildest stage, when it is just beginning to affect a person's functioning, to the most severe stage, when the person must depend completely on others for basic activities of daily living. The causes of dementia can vary, depending on the types of brain changes that may be taking place.

Other dementias include Lewy body dementia, frontotemporal disorders, and vascular dementia. It is common for people to have mixed dementia—a combination of two or more disorders, at least one of which is dementia. For example, some people have both Alzheimer's disease and vascular dementia.

Alzheimer's disease is named after Dr. Alois Alzheimer. In 1906, he noticed changes in the brain tissue of a woman who had died of an unusual mental illness. Her symptoms included memory loss, language problems, and unpredictable behavior. Dr. Alzheimer

---

6 https://www.nia.nih.gov/health/alzheimers-disease-fact-sheet

found many abnormal clumps (now called amyloid plaques) and tangled bundles of fibers (now called neurofibrillary, or tau, tangles) in the woman's brain. These plaques and tangles in the brain are still considered some of the main features of Alzheimer's disease. Another feature is the loss of connection between nerve cells (neurons) in the brain. Neurons transmit messages between different parts of the brain, and from the brain to muscles and organs in the body.

Early Symptoms:[7]

- Forgetting important things, particularly newly learned information or important dates
- Asking for the same information again and again
- Trouble solving basic problems, such as keeping track of bills or following a favorite recipe
- Losing track of the date or time of year
- Losing track of where they are and how they got there
- Trouble with depth perception or other vision problems
- Trouble joining conversations or finding the right word for something
- Misplacing things and not being able to retrace their steps to find them
- Increasingly poor judgment
- Withdrawal from work and social situations
- Changes in mood and personality

Later Symptoms:[8]

- Severe mood swings and behavior changes
- Deepening confusion about time, place, and life events
- Suspicions about friends, family, or caregivers
    - Trouble speaking, swallowing, or walking
    - Severe memory loss

Early onset Alzheimer's disease[9] is the most common form of dementia, usually affecting older adults, but it can also affect people in their 30s and 40s. When Alzheimer's disease occurs in someone under age 65, it is known as early onset (or younger-onset)

---

7 https://www.hopkinsmedicine.org/healthlibrary/conditions/nervous_system_disorders/early onset_alzheimers_disease_134,63
8 IBID
9 IBID

Alzheimer's disease. Very few people with Alzheimer's disease have the early onset form. Early onset Alzheimer's progresses faster than standard Alzheimer's disease.

Experts don't know what triggers the start of Alzheimer's disease. They suspect that two types of proteins damage and kill nerve cells. Fragments of one protein, beta-amyloid, build up and are called plaques. Twisted fibers of another protein, tau, are called tangles. Almost everyone develops plaques and tangles as they age. But those with Alzheimer's disease develop many, many more.

At first, these plaques and tangles damage the memory areas of the brain. Over time, they affect more areas of the brain. Experts don't know why some people develop so many plaques and tangles or how they spread and damage the brain.

Family history of the disease is the only known risk factor at this time. Dominantly inherited Alzheimer's disease (DIAD)—also known as autosomal dominant Alzheimer's disease—is a form of dementia caused by rare, inherited gene mutations. A person born with one of these gene mutations not only typically develops Alzheimer's disease before the age of 60, but has a 50-50 chance of passing the mutation on to each of his or her children. The disease is identifiable through genetic testing.[10,11]

For most people with early onset Alzheimer's disease, the symptoms closely mirror those of other forms of Alzheimer's disease.

Early Symptoms:[12]

- Forgetting important things, particularly newly learned information or important dates
- Asking for the same information again and again
- Trouble solving basic problems, such as keeping track of bills or following a favorite recipe
- Losing track of the date or time of year
- Losing track of where they are and how they got there

---

10 https://dian.wustl.edu/about/what-is-diad/

11 https://www.nih.gov/news-events/news-releases/data-sharing-uncovers-five-new-risk-genes-alzheimers-disease. Current research indicates that in addition to confirming the known association of 20 genes with risk of Alzheimer's and identifying five additional Alzheimer's associated genes…[t]he pathway analysis implicated the immune system, lipid metabolism, and amyloid precursor protein (APP) metabolism. Mutations in the APP gene have been shown to be directly related to early onset Alzheimer's.

12 https://www.hopkinsmedicine.org/healthlibrary/conditions/nervous_system_disorders/early onset_alzheimers_disease_134,63

- Trouble with depth perception or other vision problems
- Trouble joining conversations or finding the right word for something
- Misplacing things and not being able to retrace their steps to find them
- Increasingly poor judgment
- Withdrawal from work and social situations
- Changes in mood and personality

Later Symptoms:[13]

- Severe mood swings and behavior changes
- Deepening confusion about time, place, and life events
- Suspicions about friends, family, or caregivers
- Trouble speaking, swallowing, or walking
- Severe memory loss

My Experience

Nora, my wife, was diagnosed at 56 years old in July of 2009. However, symptoms began to show up in 2000 and 2001 when she was 47 or 48. The doctors gave her a life expectancy of four to 10 years. She was placed in a memory care center in January 2013, three-and-a-half years after diagnosis, passing away eight years and three months after diagnosis, in October of 2017.

We found out she had the defective gene when UCSF did an autopsy and DNA testing. When Nora was diagnosed, she volunteered to donate her brain and spine to UCSF for testing. When she passed, I called UCSF and they coordinated with the mortuary, took the body, extracted the brain and spine, and then returned the remains to the mortuary where she was then cremated. About seven months later, I received the autopsy report. On a conference call with me and the doctor who made the original diagnosis, was a DNA consultant. I thought this was curious, as I did not immediately understand why a DNA consultant was necessary, but Nora's doctors knew we had a daughter, Anne. The doctor explained to me that Nora had Lewy bodies as well as Alzheimer's disease and asked if I wanted a DNA test to determine if Nora had this gene defect. Before I answered, he introduced me to a DNA consultant who talked with me about the implications of DNA testing. She then asked me two questions. One I was expecting, *Do you want to know?* but the other question was a surprise and an outstanding question: *Does Anne want to know?* If Anne does not want to know, does she not want me to know if Nora had the

---

13 IBID

defective gene? A very astute observation and completely justified as to why the DNA consultant was on the call.

It never occurred to me that my knowing, if Anne didn't want to know, would be a problem. Upon reflection, I can see why it would be. Would my knowledge change my interactions with Anne? I told them that I would talk with Anne and give the DNA consultant's phone number to her if she wanted it. The result of the conversation with Anne was that she did not want to know, however, she had no objection if I knew. I called the DNA consultant and indicated that I wanted to know. In less than a month, she indicated that Nora had the defective gene and that there was a 50-50 chance that it was passed on to Anne. Anne would have to get a DNA test specifically for this gene to find out if she received it. The major issue for Anne was what she would do if she received the defective gene. Is it better to not know and see what happens, or to know and plan accordingly. If no, sigh with relief; if yes, what then? This was really difficult for Anne as she already suffers from anorexia nervosa and systemic lupus erythematosus.

Lewy body dementia[14] or dementia with Lewy body, is an umbrella term for two related clinical diagnoses

- Dementia with Lewy bodies (DLB) and
- Parkinson's disease dementia (PDD)

A diagnosis of Parkinson's disease dementia (PDD) requires a well-established diagnosis of Parkinson's that later progresses into dementia, along with very similar symptoms of DLB. A rather arbitrary time cutoff was established to differentiate between DLB and PDD

- People whose dementia occurs before or within one year of Parkinson's symptoms are diagnosed with *DLB*

- People who have an existing diagnosis of Parkinson's for more than a year and later develop dementia are diagnosed with *PDD*

The latest clinical diagnostic criteria for dementia with Lewy bodies categorize symptoms into three types, listed below.

---

14 https://www.lbda.org/go/symptoms-0

Central Features

- Progressive dementia—deficits in attention and executive function are typical
- Prominent memory impairment may not be evident in early stages

Core Features

- Fluctuating cognition with pronounced variations in attention and alertness
- Recurrent complex visual hallucinations, typically well-formed and detailed
- Spontaneous features of Parkinsonism

Suggestive Features

- REM sleep behavior disorder, which can appear years before the onset of dementia and Parkinsonism
- Severe sensitivity to neuroleptics (antipsychotic drugs) occurs in up to 50% of LBD patients
- Low dopamine transporter uptake in the brain's basal ganglia (performs a variety of functions including voluntary motor control, procedural learning relating to routine behaviors or habits such as bruxism (teeth grinding) and eye movements, as well as cognitive and emotional functions). Basal ganglia are seen on single-photon emission computed tomography (SPECT) and positron emission tomography (PET) imaging scans; both use radioisotopes to create the image

Supportive Features

- Repeated falls and syncope (fainting)
- Transient, unexplained loss of consciousness
- Autonomic dysfunction
- Hallucinations of other senses, like touch or hearing
- Visuospatial abnormalities
- Other psychiatric disturbances

LBD is the second most common dementia and usually exhibits itself in people 50 years or older. It attacks the frontal lobe first, which is why short-term memory is not affected in the early stages of this dementia. It lasts from three to eight years.

Vascular dementia,[15] occurs most often in people over 65 years as a result of strokes and lasts five to 20 years. Changes in thinking skills sometimes occur suddenly following strokes that block major brain blood vessels as well as

- Thinking problems may begin mild and worsen gradually as a result of multiple minor strokes or other conditions that affect smaller blood vessels, leading to cumulative damage

- Looks like Alzheimer's, however, there is less memory loss and more pronounced personality change

- May exhibit aggressive, abusive, and/or physical behavior

Frontotemporal disorders (FTD) is usually diagnosed in one under 60 years old and lasts seven to 13 years causing:[16,17,18]

- Degeneration in the parts of the brain that control decision-making, behavior, emotion and language (typically the frontal, temporal, and insular regions)

- Gradual and steady changes in behavior; the earliest changes typically include a disregard for social conventions, impulsivity, apathy, loss of sympathy or empathy, repetitive or compulsive movements, dietary changes, and poor insight, planning and assessment

- Gradual and steady language dysfunction—the majority of people with one of the language variants have problems expressing themselves, while their memory stays relatively intact; difficulties reading and writing develop

- Gradual and steady weakness or slowing of movement—often described as a general weakening of muscles or slowing of movements and might feel uncoordinated or like they are walking through water; they may also experience

15 https://www.alz.org/dementia/vascular-dementia-symptoms.asp
16 https://memory.ucsf.edu/frontotemporal-dementia
17 A Patient's Guide to Behavioral Variant Frontotemporal Dementia (bvFTD), UCSF Dementia Patient Guide_bvFTD_11-3-17.pdf
18 https://www.theaftd.org/what-is-ftd/disease-overview/

muscle spasms, and in neurological exams, some slowing of particular eye movements, changes in the typical reflexes and muscle stiffness or slowness may be apparent

- Saying or doing inappropriate things in social settings, displaying a lack of motivation, increased frustration, repeating sounds or movements, shoplifting, impulsively buying things, overeating, or forgetting to bathe

- Thinking problems may cause changes such as trouble focusing, paying attention, planning, making decisions, or understanding conversations; some people with FTD may have weakness in their muscles, difficulty swallowing or walking and may not recognize themselves in a mirror

Level of Care Required

25% Care
- Answering repetitive questions
- Managing the joint calendar
- Questions about their driving ability
- Bringing the family up to speed
- Dealing with denial (you, the diagnosed, family, and friends)
- Beginning to manage finances alone

50% Care
- Issues around leaving the diagnosed home by themselves
- Taking driving away
- Restricting travel and entertaining
- Coping with relations who do not want to help or get involved
- Managing when they get lost or will not stay put
- Having to speak and make choices for them
- Handling all the finances
- Communicating becomes instructional rather than conversational

75% Care
- Needing in-home care or placement as it becomes a 24/7 job
- They might be wandering
- Dressing/undressing
- Managing their eating, personal hygiene, and sleep
- May involve going into hospice
- Communicating is difficult and almost totally instructional

100% Care

- Coping with determining everything for the person
- Dealing with incontinence
- Assisting with feeding and all personal hygiene
- Giving constant attention and care
- They may become immobile or a fall risk
- Death is imminent

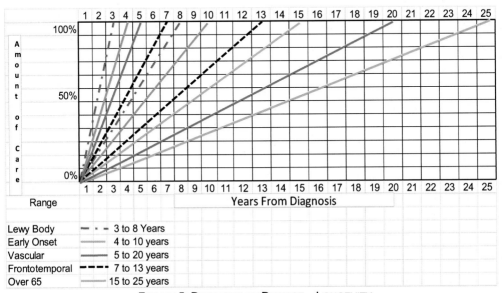

FIGURE 5: DYNAMICS OF DISEASE—LONGEVITY

This graphic emphasizes that as caregivers, we are in a multiyear process. This is not going to be a two-, three-, or six-month experience. It is going to last *years*. So, we must begin to look at how we are going to take care of ourselves so that we can survive.

CHAPTER 2: STAGES OF ALZHEIMER'S DISEASE

The "stages of the disease" are tools[19] to judge the disease's progress. I found it quite useful to understand where Nora was in the progression of the disease. This gave me some comfort as my stress increased because I did not know how long the disease process was going to be. No doctor could tell me how long; they did not know nor did they want to guess. However, knowing stages is helpful. Some authorities use **three stages** to measure progression

Mild Alzheimer's Disease (Early Stage)[20]

In the early stage of Alzheimer's, a person may function independently. He or she may still drive, work, and be part of social activities. Despite this, the person may feel as if he or she is having memory lapses, such as forgetting familiar words or the location of everyday objects.

Friends, family, or others close to the individual begin to notice difficulties. During a detailed medical interview, doctors may be able to detect problems in memory or concentration. Common difficulties include:

- Problems coming up with the right word or name
- Trouble remembering names when introduced to new people
- Challenges performing tasks in social or work settings
- Forgetting material that one has just read
- Losing or misplacing a valuable object
- Increasing trouble with planning or organizing

Moderate Alzheimer's Disease (Middle Stage)[21]

Moderate Alzheimer's is typically the longest stage and can last for many years. As the disease progresses, the person with Alzheimer's will require a greater level of care.

---

19 https://www.alz.org/alzheimers_disease_stages_of_alzheimers.asp
20 IBID
21 IBID

You may notice them confusing words, getting frustrated, angry, or acting in unexpected ways, such as refusing to bathe. Damage to nerve cells in the brain can make it difficult to express thoughts and perform routine tasks. At this point, symptoms will be noticeable to others and may include:

- Forgetfulness of events or about one's own personal history

- Feeling moody or withdrawn, especially in socially or mentally challenging situations

- Being unable to recall their own address or telephone number or the high school or college from which they graduated

- Confusion about where they are or what day it is

- The need for help choosing proper clothing for the season or the occasion

- Some trouble controlling bladder and bowels

- Changes in sleep patterns, such as sleeping during the day and becoming restless at night

- An increased risk of wandering and becoming lost

- Personality and behavioral changes, including suspiciousness and delusions or compulsive, repetitive behavior like hand-wringing or tissue shredding

Severe Alzheimer's Disease (Late Stage)[22]

In the final stage of this disease, individuals lose the ability to respond to their environment, to carry on a conversation and, eventually, to control movement. They may still say words or phrases, but communicating becomes difficult. As memory and cognitive skills continue to worsen, significant personality changes may take place and individuals need extensive help with daily activities. At this stage, individuals may:

- Need round-the-clock assistance with daily activities and personal care

- Lose awareness of recent experiences as well as of their surroundings

---

22 IBID

- Experience changes in physical abilities, including the ability to walk, sit and, eventually, swallow

- Have increasing difficulty communicating

- Become vulnerable to infections, especially pneumonia

Others authorities use **seven stages** to measure progress. I preferred the seven stages as it pinpointed where Nora was.

Stage 1—Preclinical Stage[23]
A newly defined stage, reflecting current evidence that measurable biomarker changes in the brain may occur years before symptoms affecting memory, thinking, or behavior can be detected by affected individuals or their physicians. While the guidelines identify these preclinical changes as an Alzheimer's stage, they do not establish diagnostic criteria that doctors can use now. Rather, they propose additional research to establish which biomarkers may best confirm that Alzheimer's-related changes are underway and how to measure them.

Stage 2—Very Mild Cognitive Decline[24]
The person may feel as if he or she is having memory lapses, but no symptoms of dementia can be detected during a medical examination or by friends, family, or coworkers.

Stage 3—Mild Cognitive Decline
Friends, family or coworkers begin to notice difficulties.
During a detailed medical interview, doctors may be able to detect problems in memory or concentration, such as:

- Problems coming up with the right word or name

- Trouble remembering names when introduced to new people

- Having greater difficulty performing tasks in social or work settings

- Forgetting material that one has just read

---

23 https://www.alz.org/documents/heartofamerica/Stages_of_Alzheimers.pdf
24 http://act.alz.org/site/DocServer/sevenstages.pdf?docID=16881 (Stages Two through Seven)

- Losing or misplacing a valuable object

- Increasing trouble planning or organizing

Stage 4—Moderate Cognitive Decline
A careful medical interview should be able to detect symptoms in several areas:

- Forgetfulness of recent events

- Difficulty performing complex tasks, such as planning dinner for guests, paying bills, or managing finances

- Forgetfulness about one's own personal history

- Becoming moody or withdrawn

Stage 5—Moderately Severe Cognitive Decline
Gaps in memory and thinking are noticeable, and individuals begin to need help with day-to-day activities. Individuals may:

- Be unable to recall their address or telephone number or the high school or college from which they graduated

- Become confused about where they are or what day it is but still remember significant details about themselves and their family

Stage 6—Severe Cognitive Decline
Memory continues to worsen, personality changes may take place, and individuals need extensive help with daily activities. At this stage, individuals may:

- Lose awareness of recent experiences as well as of their surroundings

- Remember their own name but have difficulty with their personal history

- Distinguish familiar and unfamiliar faces but have trouble remembering the name of a spouse or caregiver

- Need help dressing properly

- Experience major changes in sleep patterns and have trouble controlling their bladder or bowels

- Experience major personality and behavioral changes and may wander or become lost

Stage 7—Very Severe Cognitive Decline

In the final stage of the disease, individuals may lose the ability to:

- Respond to their environment
- Carry on a conversation
- Control movement
- Care for themselves, including eating or using the toilet
- Smile, sit without support, and hold their heads up
- Swallow easily; reflexes become abnormal and muscles grow rigid

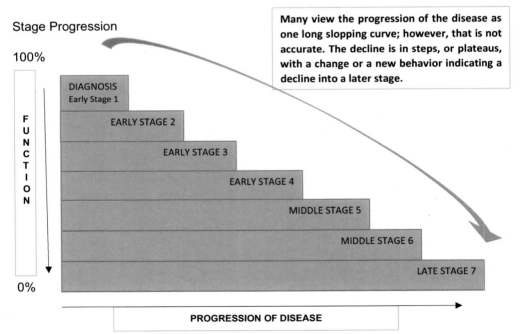

FIGURE 6: STAGES AND PROGRESSION OF THE DISEASE

I want to emphasize that the disease progresses in plateaus, or steps. We cannot predict when a new stage, plateau, or step is going to begin. As we go along in one stage, it seems overnight or without warning a new behavior starts that indicates one is entering a new stage of the disease. And it is a cumulative process; as the diagnosed moves from one stage to another, they may continue to exhibit behaviors of the previous stages.

I had so wanted it to be a slow, long, predictable slope. That was not the case and is why it is difficult to determine when certain activities or behaviors, such as driving, using power tools, etc., are no longer appropriate. We will talk more about this later.

CHAPTER 3: ALZHEIMER'S STATISTICS

It is important to know that you are not alone in being a caregiver. This chapter is a compilation of statistics about how widespread Alzheimer's disease and dementia are across my state (Oregon), nation, and world. This chapter also includes a discussion of the costs of caring for someone who has dementia and the types of resources that are available to assist the caregiver in support and financially.

People Who Have Alzheimer's Disease

- Currently, about 69,000 **Oregon**ians[25] live with Alzheimer's; about 1.7% of Oregon residents; this number is expected to increase to 84,000 by 2025

- Of 545,000 Oregonians 55 or older, 12.6% (69,000) are afflicted with Alzheimer's disease or related dementia

- Over 155,000 unpaid caregivers in Oregon provide over $5.2 billion worth of unpaid care each year—this translates to 2.2 caregivers ($155,000/$69,000) for every diagnosed patient; gives pause to the idea of one caregiver is all that is needed

- Oregon's Medicaid cost alone is about $253 million a year

  o The Medicaid cost is mostly to institutions (memory care, nursing homes, foster homes, etc.) and caregivers in the home

- Currently, about 154,000 **Virginia**ns[26] live with Alzheimer's; about 1.8% of Virginia residents; this number is expected to increase to 190,000 by 2025

- Of 1,894,605 Virginians 55 or older, 7.9% (154,000) are afflicted with Alzheimer's disease or related dementia

- Over 349,000 unpaid caregivers in Virginia provide over $7.9 billion worth of unpaid care each year—This translates to 2.2 caregivers ($349,000/$154,000) for every diagnosed patient; gives pause to the idea of one caregiver is all that is needed

- Virginia's Medicaid cost alone is about $1 billion a year

  o The Medicaid cost is mostly to institutions (memory care, nursing homes, foster homes, etc.) and caregivers in the home.

---

25 https://www.alz.org/media/Documents/oregon-alzheimers-facts-figures-2021.pdf
26 https://www.alz.org/media/Documents/virginia-alzheimers-facts-figures-2021.pdf

United States[27]

- Currently, 5.8 million Americans are living with Alzheimer's; about 1.8% of the total population (326 million) are diagnosed with Alzheimer's disease or related dementia

- Of 93.2 million Americans over 55, 6.2% are living with Alzheimer's disease or related dementia

- A little over one in 10 people age 65 and older (11.4%) have Alzheimer's disease

- Almost two-thirds of Americans with Alzheimer's are women

- Older African-Americans are about twice as likely to have Alzheimer's or other dementias as older whites

- Hispanics are about 1.5 times as likely to have Alzheimer's or other dementias as older whites

Worldwide[28]

- Currently, there are about 50 million people worldwide with dementia; about 0.6% of the world's population (7.6 billion)

- Of 617 million people over the age of 65, 8.1% have Alzheimer's disease or related dementia

- By 2030, there will be about 76 million people worldwide with dementia

Average Cost of Care

Of the total lifetime cost of caring for someone with dementia, 70% is borne by families— either through out-of-pocket health and long-term care expenses or from the value of unpaid care.

At Home

- Professional caregivers

- Generally paid hourly, can range from $12 to $40/hour

- Rate may depend on what duties the caregiver may perform, such as cooking, housekeeping, dressing, bathing, etc.

27 https://alz.org/alzheimers-dementia/facts-figures
28 https://www.alzint.org/about/dementia-facts-figures/dementia-statistics/

Hospice[29]

- General inpatient care (24-hour) is $743.55/day; $22,306.50/month; these are Medicare/Medicaid rates

- My experience was about $5,000/month, out-of-pocket, for four months of hospice care in a facility with twice-daily visits and some services such as bathing; health insurance covered a major portion of the cost

In a Facility

When a person with Alzheimer's disease and related dementias moves to a nursing home to receive 24-hour care, the financial cost to families is great; an estimated $78,000 per year.[30] The average cost of a memory care facility in Fairfax County, Virginia, is $7,016/month.[31] The lifetime cost of care for a person with Alzheimer's is around $341,840.[32]

My Experience

- Fern Gardens, a memory care facility in Medford, Oregon, cost $4,900/month, or $58,800/year

- Doctor's fees ($250/month), support materials—e.g., adult diapers, hygiene products, medications ($100/month); that comes to another $4,200/year

- Miscellaneous costs such as clothes, $1,200/year

- Total costs for my experience was $64,500/year

Nora was not eligible for Medicare because she was under 65, so this was all out-of-pocket. Her placement, from January 2013 to October 2017, totaled $310,000.

Oregon memory care facilities were cheaper than Marin County, California by $2,000 to $3,000 per month; if we had not moved, this would have added up to another $174,000/year—or $484,000 for the 58 months. Virginia's cost is an average. Note: This does not include attorney costs for guardianship, required by some memory care facilities.

---

29 https://www.cms.gov/Outreach-and-Education/Medicare-Learning-Network-MLN/MLNMattersArticles/downloads/MM10131.pdf

30 https://www.alz.org/oregon/documents/spado_report.pdf

31 https://www.caring.com/senior-living/memory-care-facilities/virginia/fairfax

32 Op. cit; (https://alz.org/facts/)

Memory Care Facility	Ashland, Fern Gardens		Marin County, CA	Virginia
	Single	Double		Approximate
Room	5200	4900	7-9,000	7016
Doctor	250	250	3-400	300
Medicines	125	125	150	150
Supplies	100	100	125	125
Total Per Month	5675	5375	7575 - 9675	7591
Total per Year	68,500	64,500	90,900 - 116,100	91,092

Full-Service Memory Care

The average stay in a memory care facility is 17 months.[33] However, there are a lot of variables in lengths of stays. To name a few:

- Type of dementia and speed of progression

- Physical condition of the person at time of placement

- Additional ailments, such as diabetes, cancer, COPD

- Stage of the disease when the person is placed (middle or late stage)

- Advance directive instructions and adherence, such as if it directs not prolonging the illness by stopping certain medications, such as insulin; Aricept; etc.

My Experience

In one of my support groups, two caregivers' spouses were over 65 when they were diagnosed with Alzheimer's disease and placed. "Dylan's" wife was in a facility for four months and passed. "Diane's" husband was in a facility and passed in a little over a year. I placed my wife, who was diagnosed with early onset Alzheimer's disease at 56, and she passed after *four years* and nine months. I had also stopped all "life-prolonging medications," such as Aricept, statins, etc., when I placed her.

Possible Sources of Caregiving Funds

- Personal wages/salary

- Investments (mutual funds, stocks, bonds: treasuries, municipals, state and corporates; money market instruments: CDs; commercial paper, T-bills)

---

33 http://www.lifecarefunding.com/white-papers/moving-into-long-term-care-facility/

- Retirement funds
- Real estate (equity in home, reverse mortgage, refinancing)
- Savings
- Family: Children can be very helpful in this process. They may help pay the cost of health care for their parents. They may even get involved in caregiving. However, complications may arise when there is a divorce and the children are associated with one spouse or the other. In some cases, the "step" children will not assist in the care of their stepmother or stepfather. Several times in facilitating a support group, I would hear about the lack of caregiver support from stepchildren. The stepchildren's interest was in the natural mother or father, not in support of the caregiver. It is unusual for relatives, such as parents, grandparents, aunts or uncles to help pay for caregiving—most of their help comes in the form of providing caregiving at no cost.
- Friends: It is uncommon for a friend of the family to financially help support the caregiving costs of the family. Most of the support from a friend is occasionally substituting for the caregiver at no cost.
- Government
  - Medicare[34] is a federal health insurance program generally for people age 65 or older who are receiving Social Security retirement benefits or who are younger than 65 and received SS disability benefits for at least 24 months
  - Medicare covers inpatient hospital care and some doctors' fees and other medical items for people with Alzheimer's or dementia who are 65 or older
  - Medicare Part D also covers many prescription drugs
  - Medicare will pay for up to 100 days of skilled nursing home care under limited circumstances. However, custodial long-term nursing home care is not covered
  - Medicare will pay for hospice care delivered in the home, a nursing facility, or an inpatient hospice facility for people with dementia determined by a doctor to be near the end of life
  - There are Medicare special needs plans (SNPs) available for individuals with dementia, Alzheimer's disease, or other chronic, terminal diseases
    - These plans are tailored to the type of chronic illness the person may have

---

34 https://www.alz.org/care/alzheimers-dementia-medicare.asp

- There are SNPs (e.g., Medicare Advantage plans) that specialize in care and coverage for beneficiaries with dementia
- Learn more information about Medicare SNPs at *https://www.medicare .gov/sign-up-change-plans/types-of-medicare-health-plans/how-medicare-special-needs-plans-snps-work.*

○ Medicaid[35] is a federal/state program typically administered by each state's welfare agency

- Eligibility and benefits vary by state. If the person with dementia is eligible for supplemental security Income (SSI), he or she usually is automatically eligible for Medicaid. Those not on SSI must have limited income and assets; the amount is determined by each state. When determining income and asset levels for individuals who live in a nursing home, there are specific guidelines to protect spouses who live in the community from impoverishment.

- Special considerations: The person with dementia should be very careful about giving away assets to family members to qualify for Medicaid. Strict laws govern this area. Check with your legal adviser to be sure you are fully aware of the legal and financial results of transferring property and wealth.

- Medicaid and long-term care: Most people with Alzheimer's disease or other dementias will eventually need long-term care services and many will require nursing home care. For people who meet eligibility requirements:
    ○ Medicaid covers all or a portion of nursing home costs
    ○ Not all nursing homes accept Medicaid
    ○ Most states have home- and community-care options for people who qualify, which allow individuals to live in their homes and receive long-term care services

To apply for Medicaid, contact your local department of welfare or department of health. Medicaid is based on financial need; you will be asked to supply information, including:

- where you live
- family members
- your monthly income

---

35 https://www.alz.org/care/alzheimers-dementia-medicaid.asp

- property
- belongings
- savings
- investments
- medical expenses

Most nursing homes that accept Medicaid have staff that can assist you in applying. *Go to Medicaid's website* for more information.

Preservation of Spousal Assets[36]

Oregon supplemental income program—medical (OSIPM) is a long-term services Medicaid program administered by the Oregon Department of Human Services. Your area may have a similar program. OSIPM provides medical coverage and long-term services for people with a low income or high long-term services expenses. For married couples, OSIPM allows one spouse to become eligible for OSIPM benefits without the other spouse becoming impoverished. What resources may each spouse keep?

---

36 https://apps.state.or.us/Forms/Served/de1999.pdf

2021 Oregon or Virginia Medicaid Long-Term Care Eligibility for Seniors[37]									
Type of Medicaid	Single			Married (both spouses applying)			Married (one spouse applying)		
	Income Limit	Asset Limit	Level of Care Required	Income Limit	Asset Limit	Level of Care Required	Income Limit	Asset Limit	Level of Care Required
Institutional / Nursing Home Medicaid	$2,382 / month*	$2,000	Nursing Home	$4,764 / month*	$4,000	Nursing Home	$2,382 / month for applicant*	$2,000 for applicant & $130,380 for non-applicant	Nursing Home
Medicaid Waivers / Home and Community-Based Services	$2,382 / month	$2,000	Nursing Home	$4,764 / month	$4,000	Nursing Home	$2,382 / month for applicant	$2,000 for applicant & $130,380 for non-applicant	Nursing Home
Regular Medicaid / Aged Blind and Disabled	$794 / month	$2,000	None	$1,191 / month	$3,000	None	$1,191 / month	3,000	None

There are two terms coupled with the word spouse: a "qualified" spouse is the one that is diagnosed or has dementia; the "community" spouse is the partner who is the caregiver.

In **Oregon**, you must complete a resource assessment form at the local office serving seniors and people with disabilities. You have to list and verify the value of all your resources at the time one spouse began receiving long-term services and at the time you apply for OSIPM long-term services. OSIPM limits the OSIPM-*qualified* spouse's resources to $2,000. The *community* spouse may keep one of the following resource amounts:

- Resources worth at least $25,284

- One-half of the total countable resources owned at the time services began if that amount is more than $25,284 but not more than $126,420, or

- More than the $126,420 maximum if your income is very low

37 https://www.medicaidplanningassistance.org/medicaid-eligibility-oregon/ and https://www.medicaidplanningassistance.org/medicaid-eligibility-virginia/

The **Virginia** Medicaid program pays for nursing home care but it also offers a "Medicaid waiver" to pay for care outside of nursing homes, called "home and community-based services" or HCBS. Virginia recently redesigned its HCBS waivers, consolidating the old elderly or disabled waiver and the technology assisted waiver into the Commonwealth Coordinated Care Plus (CCC+) waiver.

This waiver includes benefits such as adult day care, home care, and financial support to make home modifications that help residents remain in their homes. Unfortunately, unlike nursing home Medicaid which is an entitlement, CCC+ is not an entitlement program. This means CCC+ has limited enrollment, and waiting lists may exist. Furthermore, it is unclear at this point whether CCC+ would consider "assisted living" as someone's home and whether services could be provided in such a location. The same uncertainty applies to "independent living." That said, the state does offer the auxiliary grant that can be used to pay for assisted living care. Some resources do not count, including the home in which either spouse lives, a car, a burial plot, and a limited burial plan.

It is a very complicated and confusing process. It is best to have a lawyer assist you in applying for this assistance.

Professional Caregivers

An **in-home care**[38] agency is primarily engaged in providing in-home care services for compensation to an individual in their place of residence. In-home care agencies are not home health agencies; they do not provide home health services as defined in ORS 443.005:

> In-home care services are personal care services furnished by an in-home care agency, or an individual under an arrangement or contract with an in-home care agency that are necessary to assist an individual in meeting the individual's daily needs, but do not include curative or rehabilitative services.

You must become licensed as an in-home care agency if you are doing one or more of the following: scheduling caregivers, assigning work or compensation rates, defining working conditions, negotiating for a caregiver or client for the provision of services, or placing a caregiver with a client. Types of services that in-home care agencies provide include but are not limited to

---

38 http://www.oregon.gov/DHS/SENIORS-DISABILITIES/PROVIDERS-ARTNERS/LTCCN/Documents/04082015%20LTCCN%20Policy%20for%20Providers_Slides%20Only.pdf

Bathing, personal grooming and hygiene, dressing, toileting and elimination, mobility and movement, nutrition/hydration and feeding, housekeeping tasks, laundry tasks, shopping and errands, transportation, and arranging for medical appointments

In-home care agencies may also provide medication and nursing services, but these services require additional conditions for approval. These conditions include additional policies and procedures, and a nurse on staff.

Social Workers[39]

One aspect all of social work has in common is the intake or initial examination of both a client and their situation. This occurs at many levels, from the intuitive to the thorough analysis of data that a client will provide. In the case of social work in a medical or counseling environment, this can take the form of diagnosis of mental conditions that are noticeable in the way the client presents.

This can also take the form of a careful evaluation of a client's economic background in the case of a family support worker trying to determine a family's eligibility for government assistance. The initial evaluation of a client during the intake process is the first point of contact and allows the social worker to get their bearings to better serve the client.

When a client is in crisis, the social worker's job is to effectively evaluate both the client and their current situation. This kind of analysis helps the social worker to understand what intervention will be most effective to aid the client.

Sometimes, it is simply a matter of connecting a client with resources such as government assistance in order to stabilize a situation that is purely economic in nature. In other cases, a client might be in need of medical or mental health care.

Social work can also take on the form of acting in a counseling capacity. This can be as a mental health counselor (commonly called a licensed clinical social worker, or LCSW), or a substance abuse/addictions counselor.

In all of these forms, the goal of the social worker is to empower the client to see and build their own inner strengths so that they can overcome the challenges they are facing in their lives.

---

39 https://www.humanservicesedu.org/definition-social-work.html

Personal Consultants/Social Workers

Most personal consultants are trained social workers or psychologists. From what I saw and from facilitating caregiver support groups, the consultants usually represent the person diagnosed with dementia/Alzheimer's disease.

They become the care receiver's advocate and work with the caregiver to aid and care for the diagnosed. They are compensated or there is a consultant fee associated with their work.

Examples of Personal Consultants

OREGON

- *Power of the Heart: Dementia Care Education and Behavior Coaching!* (Marya Kain [40]) "While a diagnosis and a basic understanding of the brain and the illnesses is important, and indeed fascinating, my life work is about meeting the person underneath the manifestations of the illness(es) that contribute to their dementia symptoms. It is here that we can connect to build a life worth living. By getting to know who a person is and what is important to them, we can truly partner with them to help them have a meaningful life, focusing on the value of each moment."

- *Anam Cara Center for Learning and Care, The Memory Care Project* (Elizabeth V. Hallett Consulting[41]) "I specialize in dementia care education and guidance for families living with memory loss. This can include a person experiencing early dementia as well as their family members. It can also be support for caregivers as the dementia of a friend or family member progresses. I also work as the director of The Memory Care Project, a nonprofit in Southern Oregon devoted to support and education for those living with dementia in the family."

VIRGINIA

- *Elder Care Consultants*[42] "Providing dementia education and care is one of the most challenging and rewarding areas of expertise for our team. We understand the options for providing care and the costs and challenges associated with those options … We take a person-centered care approach, a philosophy of care built around the needs of

---

40 http://poweroftheheart.com/

41 https://www.linkedin.com/in/elizabeth-hallett-985691a

42 https://www.eldercc.com/care-management/dementia-education-and-care-consulting/

the individual. Person-centered care is the underlying philosophy of the Alzheimer's Association Dementia Care Practice Recommendations."

- *Lionheart Eldercare and Consulting*[43] "We never forget that everyone has unique emotions and values. We support you in making important decisions about your life, calmly and effectively. We let you know what your options are so that you are in charge. We assess each individual situation to identify resources that will create and maintain an engaging and comfortable living environment."

Hospice[44]

Hospice offers medical care toward a different goal: maintaining or improving quality of life for someone whose illness, disease, or condition is unlikely to improve. Each patient's individualized care plan is updated as needed to address the physical, emotional, and spiritual pain that often accompanies terminal illness. Hospice care also offers practical support for the caregiver(s) during the illness and grief support after the death. Hospice is something more available to the patient and the entire family when curative measures have been exhausted and life prognosis is six months or less.

The vast majority of hospices follow Medicare requirements to provide the following, as necessary, to manage the illness for which someone receives hospice care:

- Time and services of the care team, including visits to the patient's location by the hospice physician, nurse, medical social worker, home health aide and chaplain/spiritual adviser
- Medication for symptom control or pain relief
- Medical equipment like wheelchairs or walkers and medical supplies like bandages and catheters
- Physical and occupational therapy
- Speech-language pathology services
- Dietary counseling
- Any other Medicare-covered services needed to manage pain and other symptoms related to the terminal illness as recommended by the hospice team
- Short-term inpatient care (e.g., when adequate pain and symptom management cannot be achieved in the home setting)
- Short-term respite care (temporary relief from caregiving to avoid burnout)
- Grief and loss counseling for patient and loved ones

---

43 https://www.lionhearteldercare.com/caremanagement
44 https://hospicefoundation.org/Hospice-Care/Hospice-Services

What's Not Covered?

Not all services provided to patients enrolled in hospice care are covered by the Medicare hospice benefit. The benefit will **not** pay for:

- Treatment intended to cure terminal illness or unrelated to that illness
- Prescription drugs to cure illness or unrelated to that illness
- Room and board in a nursing home or hospice residential facility
- Care in an emergency room, inpatient facility care, or ambulance transportation, unless it is arranged by the hospice team or is related to the terminal illness

Family and Friends[45]

Family and friends make up the highest percentage of unpaid caregivers in the United States; 83% of the help provided to older adults in the United States comes from family members, friends, or other unpaid caregivers. Nearly half of all caregivers who provide help to older adults do so for someone with Alzheimer's or another form of dementia.

About 34% or caregivers are age 65 or older, and approximately two-thirds are women. More specifically, over one-third of dementia caregivers are daughters. The "sandwich generation" comprises approximately one-quarter of dementia caregivers not only caring for an aging parent, but also for children under the age of 18.

Alzheimer's takes a devastating toll on caregivers.[46] Compared with those caring for people without dementia, twice as many caregivers of those with dementia indicate substantial emotional, financial, and physical difficulties. According to a report from the National Consensus Development Conference on Caregiving, the most common psychological symptoms of caregiver syndrome are depression, anxiety, and anger.

Peter Vitaliano, a professor of geriatric psychiatry at the University of Washington and an expert on caregiving, said that the chronic stress of caring for someone can lead to high blood pressure, diabetes, and a compromised immune system. In severe cases, caregivers can take on the symptoms of the person that they care for; a person caring for someone with dementia may develop progressive memory loss. Worse still, this syndrome can lead to death.[47]

---

45 https://www.alz.org/facts/

46 https://www.brmmlaw.com/70-of-all-caregivers-over-the-age-of-70-die-first-is-caregiver-syndrome-a-real-medical-diagnosis/

47 IBID

My Experience

One of the facilitators of the support group was developing severe medical problems with high blood pressure and the stress of caregiving. It was readily apparent to the others in the support group that he was not doing well. We kept telling him that he had to place his wife, however, his view was that he was "handling it." Finally, his children said "if you do not place Mom, we will."

Caregiving Statistics

A Stanford University study reports that 41% of Alzheimer's disease caregivers die from stress-related disorders before the patient dies.[48] And caregivers have a 63% higher mortality rate than non-caregivers. This means that four out of 10 caregivers for Alzheimer's disease pass before the person they're caring for.

The table below shows the effects of caregiving for Oregon and Virginia and the average for the US.

STATE	Caregivers		
	With chronic health conditions	With depression	In poor physical health
Oregon	53.7%	19.9%	16.7%
Virginia	60.4%	23.6%	13.8%
US	57.5%	24.4%	13.0%

Table developed from Alzheimer's website's (alz.org) facts and figures.

Mortality Statistics

According to the report by researchers at the CDC (Centers for Disease Control) and Georgia State University, 93,541 people died from Alzheimer's in the United States in 2014, a 54.5% increase over 1999 figures.[49] Only recently have doctors and medical personnel have been listing Alzheimer's disease as a cause of death—they used to report pneumonia as cause of death, a result of Alzheimer's disease/dementia, understating the cause of death due to Alzheimer's.

---

48 https://www.nextavenue.org/caregiver-sicker-loved-one/
49 https://www.scientificamerican.com/article/u-s-alzheimers-deaths-jump-54-percent-more-dying-at-home/

During that period, the percentage of people who died from Alzheimer's in a medical facility/hospital fell by more than half, from 14.7% in 1999 to 6.6% in 2014. Meanwhile, researchers reported in the CDC's weekly report on death and disease the number of people with Alzheimer's who died at home increased to 24.9% in 2014 from 13.9% in 1999. The remainder passed under hospice care (42%) or in non-medical facilities (28%), such as foster homes or memory care.[50]

Ombudsmen[51]

The long-term care ombudsman[52] is an independent state agency that serves long-term care facility residents through complaint investigation, resolution and advocacy for improvement in resident care.

The vision of the Oregon long-term care ombudsman is that citizens living in nursing facilities, residential care facilities, assisted living facilities and adult foster care homes deserve quality care. They should enjoy freedom from abuse and neglect and the freedom to make choices about their care.

The mission of Oregon's long-term care ombudsman program is to protect individual rights, enhance quality of life, improve care, and promote dignity of residents living in Oregon's licensed long-term care facilities.

Program staff works with a statewide network of over 180 volunteers who work in their own communities in a variety of roles to achieve this vision and mission.

- The services of the long-term care ombudsman program are free and available to residents, families, facility staff, and the general public
- Ombudsmen respond to a wide variety of resident concerns, including problems with resident care, medications, billing, lost property, meal quality, evictions, guardianships, dignity and respect, and care plans
- The program serves residents in nursing facilities, residential care facilities, assisted living facilities, continuing care facilities, and adult foster care homes
- Complaints are investigated and resolved by staff and trained and certified volunteer ombudsmen assigned to facilities throughout the state

---

50 https://www.forbes.com/sites/howardgleckman/2013/02/06/more-people-are-dying-at-home-and-in-hospice-but-they-are-also-getting-more-intense-hospital-care/
51 https://www.oltco.org/ltco/about-us
52 https://www.oltco.org/programs/opg-about-us.html

- Beyond complaint investigation and resolution, ombudsmen strive to be the eyes and ears of residents and to advocate for improvements in their quality of life and quality of care
- The program also provides hundreds of free consultations each year to individuals struggling with the complexities of the long-term care system

The Residential Facilities Ombudsman (RFO) program[53] in Oregon provides advocacy services on behalf of more than 8,200 individuals living in more than 2,300 licensed or certified homes for intellectual and/or developmental disabilities as well as homes for mental health conditions statewide.

- The RFO opened its program and began visiting homes in eastern Oregon counties July of 2016; to date, they have visited 100% of homes in more than 16 counties, providing community outreach introducing the program at the same time responding to requests for assistance from virtually every county in the state
- Their goal in 2018/19 was to visit 100% of the homes in eight additional counties, respond to all requests for assistance as well as develop, recruit and train an initial group of volunteer certified ombudsman in select communities
- This initial group of volunteers will provide a foundation of training and support that they will be able to grow to every area of the state
- When they are not visiting individuals in their homes and opening services to new areas of the state they are conducting community outreach, giving presentations
- They also work with state and local offices towards improving systems as well as share recommendations with the legislature
- The Residential Facilities Ombudsman program (RFO) is part of an independent state agency that is resident rights and client-driven
- Their services are free and confidential

The Oregon Public Guardian and Conservator Program[54] serves as court-appointed, surrogate decision-makers for adults incapable of making some or most of the decisions needed to be safe due to significant cognitive impairment.

The OPGC only serves in this role as a last resort. Where guardianship is the only option to make the person safe, OPGC will become involved only if there is no other responsible person willing and able to serve.

---

53 https://www.oltco.org/programs/rfo-about-us.html
54 https://www.oltco.org/programs/opg-about-us.html

Those in need of OPG's services include persons with age-related cognitive impairment, persons who have suffered traumatic brain injuries, persons with serious and persistent mental health issues and persons with intellectual/developmental disabilities.

Guardianship is one of the most severe restrictions on a person's right to self-determination and should never be taken lightly. Under guardianship, a person loses the right to make their own decisions about their lives. A guardian has the authority to determine where someone lives, what services they receive, who their doctor is, what medical care and procedures they receive, how their income is spent, who may visit them, and many other decisions that most people take for granted.

Guardianship should only be considered as an option if all other less restrictive alternatives have been attempted and failed, or evaluated to be non-viable.

The Virginia long-term care ombudsman[55] advocates for older persons receiving long-term care services, whether provided in a nursing home or assisted living facility, or through community-based services to assist persons still living at home. They provide older Virginians, their families, and the public with information, advocacy, and assistance to help resolve care problems of individual residents and groups of residents to bring about changes at the local, state, and national levels to improve care and quality of life. The cornerstone of this work is residents' rights. While many people receive good long-term care services, others encounter problems and neglect. Ombudsmen, both paid staff and volunteers, provide help and a voice for those that are not heard or unable to speak for themselves.

The ombudsman program also has advocates that assist individuals who are participants in (CCC+). Medicaid Managed Care Advocates help to resolve problems with plan coverage, assessing plan benefits, health care, behavioral health care and long-term care services and supports. The long-term care ombudsman state agency also covers residential facilities (foster homes, residential home, etc.).

Virginia has a similar program: the Public Guardian and Conservator Program Virginia.[56] The state has the capability of selecting a guardian or conservator or both when an individual, such as the person diagnosed with Alzheimer's or dementia has no one capable or wanting to become their guardian or conservator. Virginia's program states:

---

55 https://elderrightsva.org/
56 https://law.lis.virginia.gov/admincode/title22/agency30/chapter70/section30/

A. Designation. The department shall select public guardian programs in accordance with the requirements of the Virginia Public Procurement Act. Only those programs that contract with the department shall be designated as public guardian programs. Funding for public guardian programs is provided by the appropriation of general funds.

B. Authority. A public guardian program appointed as a guardian, a conservator, or both as a guardian and conservator, shall have all the powers and duties specified in Chapter 20 (§ 64.2-2000 et seq.) of Title 64.2 of the Code of Virginia, except as otherwise specifically limited by a court.

...

E. Appointments.

1. Prior to the public guardian program accepting an individual for services, the multidisciplinary panel described in subdivision C 2 of this section shall screen referrals to ensure that:

a. The public guardian program is appointed as guardian, or conservator, or both only in those cases where guardianship or conservatorship is the least restrictive alternative available to assist the individual

b. The appointment is consistent with serving the type of client identified by the established priorities of the public guardian program

c. The individual cannot adequately care for himself

d. The individual is indigent, and

e. There is no other proper or suitable person or entity to serve as guardian.

f. In the case of an individual who receives case management services from a community services board (CSB) or behavioral health authority (BHA), the multidisciplinary panel may also request the results of the "determination of capacity" as authorized by 12VAC35-115-145 (Determination of capacity to give consent or authorization) and verification that no other person is available or willing to serve as guardian pursuant to 12VAC35-115-146 E (Authorized representatives).

2. Appointments by a circuit court shall name the public guardian program, rather than an individual person, as the guardian, the conservator or both guardian and conservator.

3. A public guardian program shall only accept appointments as guardian, conservator, or both guardian and conservator that generate no fee or that generate a minimal fee. *https://law.lis.virginia.gov/admincode/title22/agency30/chapter70/section30/*

The thing to note here is, like Oregon, Virginia's court appoints the department/agency, not an individual. It is the responsibility of the department/agency to act as a guardian and/or conservator for the person diagnosed with Alzheimer's disease or other dementias.

CHAPTER 4: DIAGNOSIS

The person developing Alzheimer's disease or dementia begins to suspect that something is wrong before anyone else does. It is usually little things, like forgetting an appointment or what day it is or being unable to figure something out, such as developing a project plan or redesigning a room or business lobby.

My Experience

Nora was the head of a local library in Marin County, California, and knew something was wrong in the early 2000s when she could not figure out how to configure the library reference desk. This moved her to resign as head librarian of the branch; it took her coworkers and management by surprise. We did not know at the time that she was exhibiting the effects of early onset Alzheimer's disease.

A word of caution. Many people think little memory lapses mean they are getting Alzheimer's disease or dementia, but it may just be typical age-related changes. Frequent memory loss that disrupts daily life may be a symptom of dementia as brain disease that causes a slow decline in memory, thinking, and reasoning skills.

Warning Signs and Symptoms

There are 10 main warning signs to look for.[57] Individuals experiencing one or more of these should see a doctor.

1. **Memory loss that disrupts daily life**

   One of the most common signs of Alzheimer's is memory loss, especially forgetting recently learned information. Other signs include forgetting important dates or events; asking for the same information over and over; increasingly needing to rely on memory aids (e.g., reminder notes or electronic devices) or family members for things they used to handle on their own.
   A typical age-related change is sometimes forgetting names or appointments but remembering them later.

---

57 https://www.alz.org/10-signs-symptoms-alzheimers-dementia.asp

2. Challenges in planning or solving problems

Some people may experience changes in their ability to develop and follow a plan or work with numbers. They may have trouble following a familiar recipe or keeping track of monthly bills. They may have difficulty concentrating and take much longer to do things than they did before.

A typical age-related change is making occasional errors when balancing a checkbook.

3. Difficulty completing familiar tasks at home, at work, or at leisure

People with Alzheimer's often find it hard to complete tasks like driving to a familiar location, managing a budget at work, or remembering the rules of a favorite game.

A typical age-related change is occasionally needing help to use the settings on a microwave or to record a television show.

4. Confusion with time or place

People with Alzheimer's can lose track of dates, seasons, and the passage of time. They may have trouble understanding something if it is not happening *right now*. Sometimes they may forget where they are or how they got there.

A typical age-related change is getting confused about the day of the week but figuring it out later.

5. Trouble understanding visual images and spatial relationships

For some people, difficulty reading, judging distance, and determining color or contrast, which may cause problems with driving.

A typical age-related change is vision changes related to cataracts.

6. New problems with words in speaking or writing

People with Alzheimer's may have trouble following or joining a conversation. They may repeat themselves or stop in the middle of a conversation and have no idea how to continue. They may struggle with vocabulary, have problems finding the right word, or call things by the wrong name (e.g., calling a watch a "hand-clock").

A typical age-related change is sometimes having trouble finding the right word.

7. Misplacing things and losing the ability to retrace steps

A person with Alzheimer's disease may put things in unusual places. They may lose things and be unable to go back over their steps to find them again. They may accuse others of stealing. This may occur more frequently over time.

A typical age-related change is misplacing things from time to time and retracing steps to find them.

8. Decreased or poor judgment

People with Alzheimer's may experience changes in judgment or decision-making. For example, giving large amounts of money to telemarketers. They may pay less attention to grooming or keeping themselves clean.

A typical age-related change is making a bad decision once in a while.

9. Withdrawal from work or social activities

A person with Alzheimer's may start to remove themselves from hobbies, social activities, work projects, or sports. They may have trouble keeping up with a favorite sports team or remembering how to complete a favorite hobby. They may also avoid being social because of the changes they have experienced.

A typical age-related change is sometimes feeling weary of work, family and social obligations.

10. Changes in mood and personality

The mood and personalities of people with Alzheimer's can change. They can become confused, suspicious, depressed, fearful, or anxious. They may be easily upset at home, at work, with friends, or wherever they are out of their comfort zone.

A typical age-related change is developing very specific ways of doing things and becoming irritable when a routine is disrupted.

Differences Between Alzheimer's and Typical Age-Related Changes

Signs of Alzheimer's/dementia	Typical age-related changes
Poor judgment and decision-making	Making a bad decision once in a while
Inability to manage a budget	Missing a monthly payment
Losing track of the date or the season	Forgetting which day it is but remembering later
Difficulty having a conversation	Sometimes forgetting which word to use
Misplacing things; unable to retrace steps	Losing things from time to time

Get the Diagnosis!

What type of dementia a person has will make a difference in understanding, coping with, and finding the level of medical support required. Each will have its own set of stresses, coping skills, progression, and behaviors. Recall our earlier session on the different types of dementia:

- Standard Alzheimer's disease
- Early onset Alzheimer's disease
- Lewy body
- Frontotemporal
- Vascular

There are several cumulative ways for a doctor to make a diagnosis of Alzheimer's or dementia, usually through eliminating other causes, such as brain tumor, physical trauma, etc. Sometimes the physician will do a quick oral test using a set question.[58] In support groups, some have indicated passing these tests, yet still insisted that something was wrong. If the person fails the quick test, the physician may recommend one or more of the following tests:

- Neuro-psychological testing (written) can take up to several hours over two days
- Brain scans (C-scan or MRI)
- Checking for beta-amyloid in the spinal fluid—if over a certain level, indicates a high correlation with Alzheimer's disease

My Experience

In 2008, after insisting for several months that something was wrong and her brain was not working right, Nora was psychologically tested by a neuro-psychologist. The test was around six to eight hours and took two days. The first result was a diagnosis of mild cognitive impairment (MCI). The medical professionals met with us and indicated that this may not lead to Alzheimer's disease.

At her very strong insistence, Nora was retested in 2009 after elimination of all other possible causes. She had blood tests and a brain scan. The psychological memory test results showed a decline in performance. Not finding any other cause, it was a diagnosis

---

58 I have found that the quick in-office test is not very reliable and I am not in favor of it. It may be useful in a few circumstances where the person is in the middle or late stages of dementia; however, if a person is saying there is something wrong and others are doubting them, this test is not useful. One needs a full neuro-psychological test which tests for a wide range of dementia dimensions.

of Alzheimer's disease and, because of her age (56), the doctor said it was early onset Alzheimer's disease. He also indicated that the typical life span was four to 10 years and that the disease moved faster than standard Alzheimer's disease. He suggested that she begin taking Aricept, a drug that slows down the progression of the disease.

Reactions to Diagnosis

When the formal diagnosis is made, there are multiple reactions possible. You need time to digest the results. It will be a shock, because it is official. It is confirmation of knowing something was wrong. You then begin to ponder *Am I embarrassed? Do I hide it? Do I talk about it?* Your reaction will be determined, in part, by your history, relationship, empathy, and compassion:

- History—How you reacted in the past to bad medical news about others, especially those close to you
- Relationship—How healthy the relationship is will influence reactions
- Empathy—Your ability to understand how the other person might feel and react
- Compassion—Your ability to be understanding and concerned for the person, *as well as for yourself*

Reactions can include sadness, fear, anger, hostility, "why me?" and/or denial. These emotions are quite normal and are not unexpected but should not last a long time or become overwhelming. If they do, seeing a therapist can help one cope with the emotions they are feeling—whether the person diagnosed or the caregiver.

My Experience

We experienced all these emotions and then sought out a therapist to help both of us to cope with this. I learned that many of my reactions and thoughts about this were due to my upbringing and how I reacted to significant, sad events in my life. It helped me to understand and to deal with my wife having a terminal illness. Nora was already seeing a therapist and was dealing with anger issues about the diagnosis as well as resentment that no one believed her when she said "something is wrong with me."

Need to Talk

You need to discuss the situation with your partner/spouse/children; with the primary *caregiver and/or the diagnosed*. Both the diagnosed partner and the future caregiver need to ask themselves and each other: *How do you feel about this?* You need to be honest.

As the caregiver, ask, *What do you want me to do for you?* to begin understanding the feelings and thoughts of the diagnosed. They may not want you to do anything, but this would be a "heat of the moment" reaction.

Ask, *What scares you the most?* What the diagnosed partner foresees may not be realistic. Then tell them what scares you the most. This lets the diagnosed understand your feelings about this.

Ask, *What things do we want to do while we can?* This is a good discussion point. In one of my support groups, a couple received the diagnosis that the wife has dementia, probably Alzheimer's. She wanted to go to Paris before she was no longer able to, so armed with this, her spouse planned a trip to Paris while she was still able to negotiate the hazards of international travel.

If, there is denial that anything is wrong in this open discussion, or *I do not see any reason to change*, or one or both of you are not able to discuss your feelings, then it behooves you both to see a therapist. Denial has become the only response to the diagnosis.

I recommend that each of you see a therapist individually. You need the privacy of expressing your true emotions without fear of hurting the other person's feelings.

My Experience

I sought out a therapist to help me deal with my feelings, reactions, and my behavior (in many cases, it was the result of how I reacted to similar situations in my life, especially in my formative years). I wanted to learn how to cope with those feelings so I could be a better caregiver. A therapist is a reality check on how you are coping with the situation.

A person in one support group did not want to place the care receiver in a memory care facility because they (the caregiver) did not want to come home to an empty house. It turns out, being a "latch-key kid" as a child was impacting their decision-making. However, their overt reason was that they felt guilty they were "pushing" the other person away.

You also need to understand that the dementia process will be a long, extended mourning period. The person before your eyes slowly recedes, becoming someone that is not the person you fell in love with, married, and/or partnered with, nor the father or mother you knew. That person becomes a memory which will be hard to deal with because they will still be physically there. You will go through most of the steps of the mourning process before they pass away. We will deal with this in more detail in Chapter 6.

Chapter 5: First Steps

After the initial shock has dissipated, the hard work begins. Three major issues need to be discussed and agreed upon: finances, legal matters, and end of life choices.

Financial Matters

In my opinion, you should open a trust. You need to move assets, debts, and policies into a trust and out of both the care receiver's and caregiver's names. This includes:

- Assets
    - Car, RVs, boats, motorcycles, etc.
    - Home(s)
    - Investments (stocks, bonds, mutual funds, property)
    - Personal effects that have value, such as jewelry, paintings
- Debts
    - Car loans
    - Home mortgage(s), home equity loans
    - Secured and unsecured loans
- Insurance policies
    - Property insurance
    - Life insurance
    - Car insurance

You will need to remove the care receiver's name from financial instruments, which may be the most difficult thing to do.

Debit and Credit Cards

You may have to take the cards away, because you usually cannot take their name off a bank account without closing it. I found out that Nora could not say "no" to any charity caller. She donated hundreds of dollars to charities that called.

I found out that you cannot remove a joint user from credit card accounts unless they agree in writing. A person in one support group had a novel solution—just close the account/card and open a totally new one with only themselves authorized. I found that too many entities had my credit card info, which would have made it very difficult and time-consuming to change them all. Our credit card issuer demanded Nora's authorization to remove her name, but it was too late when I found this out, so I just took the card away.

Beneficiaries

Change your beneficiaries to a trust where possible. This seemingly simple task can produce difficulties—I could not remove Nora as a beneficiary and name the Harris Family Trust as beneficiary without her formal consent for my deferred compensation account.[59] Nora was not capable of understanding what she was signing. Oregon state law required a court order to change the beneficiary. So, I had to get a decree to legally change the beneficiary into my name because they would not accept the trust as beneficiary.

Review Insurance Policies

You need to review healthcare insurance and long-term care insurance policies to see what the coverage is, what limitations are imposed, and who the beneficiary is.

Medicare

If you are 65 or over, you need to review what Medicare pays for, and more importantly, what it does not. You also need to review any supplemental health insurance policies: What does it cover (as far as dementia is concerned)? What does it not cover? And what is your financial obligation under their coverage, such as memory care facilities?

Health Insurance

If you are under 65, do you have health insurance? If so, you need to review your policy to determine what it covers (regarding dementia). Many policies will not cover the cost of a memory care facility, but will cover the cost of doctors and medications. If you do not have health insurance, then you need to go to the health insurance exchanges in your state or the federal government and get a policy. Dementia is not a cheap disease.

---

59 When they gave bonuses when I worked at Wells Fargo, we had a choice of receiving it now or "deferring" it to a later time, but no longer than 10 years. The payout could be in increments/payments or in a lump sum.

Long-Term Care Insurance[60]

Long-term care insurance is specifically designed to pay for the care required when a person has been diagnosed with a long-term or terminal disease. The later stages of the illness usually requires 24/7 care by professionals. This could be in a facility, such as assisted living, nursing home, memory care, hospital, etc. Usually, a daily rate is selected at the time of buying the policy, such as $100 or $250/day along with a period of time, such as 90 or 180 days.

Do you have long-term care insurance? Is it a family policy or individual? You need to review the policy for what it does and does not cover.

My Experience

I thought I had long-term care insurance since I signed up for it when I joined Wells Fargo in the mid-1990s. I bought the family policy, I thought. When Nora was diagnosed, I went over the policy and noticed in the fine print (in a footnote) that for Nora to be covered she needed to apply separately to the insurance company for approval or acceptance. I called the insurance company and they confirmed that she was not covered. I missed this requirement when I got the policy particulars. And since she was diagnosed, I was positive that she would be refused if she applied (in 2009). So, the policy was of no value for Nora's Alzheimer's diagnosis and future placement in a memory care facility.

Changing the beneficiary's name from the care receiver to a trust or to the caregiver's can be a sensitive issue. These discussions may take some time and the care receiver will need reassurance that they are not being dismissed, abandoned, or losing their independence.

Legal Matters

You will need to see a lawyer to create a trust for the financial tasks listed above and/or removing beneficiary name from financial legal documents and forms. You will need to discuss the types of trusts with the lawyer to see which one will best fit your needs. There

---

60 Long-term care refers to a host of services that aren't covered by regular health insurance, such as assistance with routine daily activities like bathing, dressing, or getting in and out of bed. A long-term care insurance policy helps cover the costs of that care for a chronic medical condition, a disability, or a disorder such as Alzheimer's disease. Most policies will reimburse for care given in a variety of places, such as your home, a nursing home, an assisted living facility, or an adult day care center. Considering long-term care costs is an important part of any long-range financial plan, especially in your 50s and beyond. **Waiting until you need care to buy coverage is not an option. You won't qualify for long-term care insurance if you already have a debilitating condition** [emphasis added]. https://www.nerdwallet.com/blog/insurance/long-term-care-insurance/

are two basic types of trusts: revocable living and irrevocable trusts. There is also guardianship, which we will discuss later.

Revocable Trust[61]

A *revocable living trust*, living trust, or *inter vivos* trust, also known as a revocable trust, is simply a type of trust that can be changed at any time. In other words, if you have second thoughts about a provision in the trust or change your mind about who should be a beneficiary or trustee of the trust, you can modify the terms of the trust through what is called a trust amendment. Or, if you decide that you don't like anything about the trust at all, you can either revoke the entire agreement or change the entire contents through a *trust amendment and restatement.*

Why should you use a revocable living trust as part of your estate plan? For four important reasons:

1. **To plan for mental disability**. Assets held in the name of a revocable living trust at the time a person becomes mentally incapacitated can be managed by their disability trustee instead of by a court-supervised guardian or conservator.

2. **To avoid probate**. Assets held in the name of a revocable living trust at the time of a person's death will pass directly to the beneficiaries named in the trust agreement and outside of the probate process.

3. **To protect the privacy of your property and beneficiaries after you die**. By avoiding probate with a revocable living trust, your trust agreement will remain a private document and avoid becoming a public record for all the world to read. It will keep the details about your assets and estate a private family matter. Contrast this with a last will and testament that has been admitted to probate; it becomes a public court record that anyone can see and read.

4. There is life after the passing of the care receiver and **you may want to make major changes in the trust** to reflect your new situation, which may include remarriage.[62]

Irrevocable Trust[63]

---

61 https://www.thebalance.com/revocable-vs-irrevocable-trusts-3505386
62 This may be a surprising statement, but I know of two caregivers that have remarried since their spouses passed. Their new partners were members of their support groups. (I also remarried within a year of Nora passing, however, my new partner was not part of a support group.)
63 https://www.thebalance.com/revocable-vs-irrevocable-trusts-3505386

An *irrevocable trust* is simply a type of trust that can't be changed after the agreement has been signed, or is a revocable trust that, by its design, becomes irrevocable after the trust-maker dies or some other specific point in time.

Irrevocable trusts, such as irrevocable life insurance trusts, are commonly used to remove the value of property from a person's estate so that the property can't be taxed when the person dies. In other words, the person who transfers assets into an irrevocable trust is giving those assets to the trustee and beneficiaries of the trust so that the person no longer owns the assets.

Another common use for an irrevocable trust is to provide asset protection for the trust-maker and the trust-maker's family. This works in the same way that an irrevocable trust does to reduce estate taxes. By placing assets into an irrevocable trust, the trust-maker is giving up complete control and access to the trust assets and, therefore, the trust assets cannot be reached by a creditor of the trust-maker or an available resource for Medicaid planning.

Another use for an irrevocable trust is charitable estate planning, such as through a charitable remainder trust or a charitable lead trust. If the trust-maker makes the initial transfer of assets into a charitable trust while still alive, the trust-maker will receive a charitable income tax deduction in the year the transfer is made. Or, if the initial transfer of assets into a charitable trust doesn't occur until after the trust-maker's death, the trust-maker's estate will receive a charitable estate tax deduction.

A main reason to set up an irrevocable trust after a spouse's Alzheimer's diagnosis is when there are stepchildren and an issue of preserving specific assets for them. A common problem with a divorce and a subsequent remarriage is the strain between the children and the stepparent. An irrevocable trust will ensure the stepchildren receive the assets agreed upon; the trustee or trust-maker cannot change this distribution.

Guardianship vs. Conservatorship[64]

A *guardian* is appointed by a court to protect and care for the health and well-being of an incapacitated person or a minor child. A petition must be filed with the appropriate court, and notice given to all interested persons. The process may be complicated; it's advisable to consult with an attorney.

---

64 https://www.courts.oregon.gov/programs/family/guardianship-conservatorship/Pages/default.aspx

A *conservator* is a fiduciary appointed by a court to protect and conserve the assets of an incapacitated person or a minor child. The process is similar to the appointment of a guardian.

My Experience

I went to court to get guardianship and conservatorship of Nora when I placed her into a memory care facility. The process was relatively simple.

- I was given temporary guardianship of Nora while the state conducted its investigation
- I provided a doctor's statement on Nora's condition (Alzheimer's disease and incapacity)
- A court-appointed representative went to interview Nora at the facility to determine incapacity
- The person also interviewed my daughter by phone to determine if there were any objections
- They then submitted a report to the court
- Finally, a judgment was filed as acceptance of permanent guardianship

2

3

IN THE CIRCUIT COURT OF THE STATE OF OREGON

FOR THE COUNTY OF JACKSON

IN THE MATTER OF THE GUARDIANSHIP	CASE NO.: 13-017-G6
OF	
NORA ███████ HARRIS,	**LIMITED JUDGMENT APPOINTING A GUARDIAN**
PROTECTED PERSON.	

On the Petition for Appointment of a Guardian for Nora ███████ Harris, and

it appearing to the Court from the allegations of the Petition, any reports submitted,

including a Visitor's Report, and all other records and files herein that:

Appointment of a Guardian in this proceeding is necessary to promote and

protect the well-being of the Respondent. The clear and convincing evidence

further shows that:

1.   Venue is properly in this Court, and no other Court in this or any other

state has acquired jurisdiction in this matter.

2.   All Notices required by ORS 125.060 have been given to the persons

entitled to Notice.

3.   The Respondent is incapacitated and the appointment of a Guardian is

Arant & Broesder, LLC
312 South Ivy Street
Medford, OR 97501
Tel: (541) 773-1222
Fax: (541) 779-5405

Page - 1 LIMITED JUDGMENT APPOINTING A GUARDIAN

1 necessary as a means of providing continuing care and supervision of the

2 Respondent.

3   4.   The Visitor has filed a Report recommending appointment of a

4 Guardian.

5   5.   William L. Harris is qualified and suitable to act as Guardian, and has

6 accepted appointment.

7   **NOW, THEREFORE, IT IS HEREBY ORDERED AND ADJUDGED:**

8   A.   William L. Harris is appointed Guardian for Nora ███ Harris, with

9 specific authority to manage the Protected Person's finances.

10   B.   The Guardian will act as the Representative Payee for Social Security.

11   C.   Letters of Guardianship shall issue to William L. Harris.

12   **DATED** this /   day of   LJc*PL*

13

14 Circuit Court Judge

15 SUBMITTED BY:
    William L. Harris, Petitioner

16

17

18 Jason C. Broesder, OSB #992289
    Arant & Broesder, LLC
19 jason@broesderlaw.com
    Of Attorneys for Petitioner
20 S:\Office\Protective Proceedings\Guardianship\Clients\Harris\Judgment.docx

Arant & Broesder, LLC
312 South Ivy Street
Medford, OR 97501
Tel: (541) 773-1222
Fax: (541) 779-5405

Page - 2 LIMITED JUDGMENT APPOINTING A GUARDIAN

54

End of Life: Advance Directives[65]

An advance directive states the health care measures treatment a person wants if they cannot speak for themselves. It indicates whether the person wants to continue curative or life-sustaining treatment.

The advance directive should not be confused with the POLST (Portable Orders for Life-Sustaining Treatment), an Oregon form which is a medical order for the specific medical treatments you want during a medical emergency.[66] POLST forms are appropriate for individuals with a serious illness or advanced frailty, nearing the end of life.

Virginia has adopted the concept from Oregon, calling it POST (Physician Orders for Scope of Treatment).

> A POST is a physician-signed order form which communicates and puts into action treatment preferences when a patient is near the end of their life. The Virginia POST form was modeled after the Oregon POLST form which has been in use for almost 20 years …
> The POST form should be completed only after the patient (or, if the patient lacks capacity, the patient's health care agent) has an advance care planning discussion with a physician or a trained POST Advance Care Planning Facilitator (ACPF) under the direction of a physician. Patients and families interested in creating a POST form should do so through their health care provider.[67]

A person must develop the advance directive while they are able to clearly and definitively express themselves verbally, in writing, or in sign language. It must express their own free will about their health care, not anyone else's. It does not affect routine care for cleanliness and comfort which must be given whether or not there is an advance directive.

Oregon law (ORS 127.505 to 127.660 and ORS 127.995) allows people to preauthorize health care professionals to permit the natural dying process if they are medically confirmed to be in one of the conditions described in their health care instructions. However, the law does not authorize euthanasia, assisted suicide, or any overt action to end their life.

---

65 https://healthcare.oregon.gov/shiba/topics/Pages/advance-directives.aspx See appendix for Advance Directives of Oregon, Virginia, Idaho, and two from Washington.
66 http://polst.org/advance-care-planning/polst-and-advance-directives/
67 https://www.virginiapost.org/forms

Filling Out an Advance Directive

Whether you are filling the advance directive out for yourself or for the care receiver, you need to consider the following:

- Who will be my "agent" to speak for me when I am unable to communicate my wishes?
- Does this person understand my wishes?
- Do I want to be resuscitated if I stop breathing or my heart stops beating?

You will also need to think about things like assisted feeding.

- Do I want someone to feed me?
- Do I want to invoke voluntary stop eating and drinking (VSED)?

As part of this discussion, the care receiver needs to consider something else. It is not just medical treatment or quality of life; do they want to financially drain their assets and leave the caregiver with minimal or no resources? This is at the heart of the "prolong the process" discussion.

There are other things to think about in filling out an advance directive. Where does the care receiver want to die? At home? In a memory care facility? Another facility, such as hospice? Some advance directives directly ask this question.

Even though the care receiver may want to die at home, I recommend the caregiver make that determination as the end approaches. You will be under enough pressure without adding to your stress by moving the loved one home and then dealing with the comings and goings of well-wishers, while trying to take care of the person in the late stages of the disease.

The last stages of the disease usually mean that the person can do little or nothing to take care of themselves, cannot communicate, are incontinent, cannot eat without assistance or may not be able to swallow, are unable to bathe themselves, and demand a high level of physical support, such as getting into and out of bed, walking, and so on. Know that hospice personnel try to make the care receiver comfortable.

Thus, your loved one dying at home is **your** decision and depends upon how you are doing and your level of stress at the end. It really does not matter what the care receiver wishes upon diagnosis, because at the later stages of disease, they are unaware of where they are, what physical and mental state they are in, and what it really means for the caregiver.

My Experience

I was happy that Nora passed in the memory care facility, as the caregivers and hospice were better able to cope and assist Nora in her last days. She started panting about 11 a.m. I stayed with her until late afternoon and then went home. I received a call at one a.m. that she had passed.

Some people might think that I was insensitive or cruel to not be with her the whole time, but she had no idea who was with her, what was being done, or what was going on in those last 14 hours. She did not know who I was and had no long- or short-term memory. She was incapable of communicating verbally or physically. All reactions were reflexive to the body dying. The staff at the facility had been through this many times and was sympathetic and attentive. I had to come to terms with my guilt.

It was very difficult to sit there and watch her struggle to breathe, to watch her die. This person was extremely articulate, very intelligent, the most widely read person I knew—a librarian and an indexer of books—was just a body gasping for air. This was after watching the person I knew for decades shrink and disappear in those eight years before she died.

Determine What Resources Are Available

How much you will be able to afford for caregivers and, possibly, memory care facilities? Or, what assets are available for financing care? Are these assets liquid or nearly immediately available (CDs, T-bills, savings or money market accounts)? Are you or your spouse still working? Is there sufficient remaining (net) income to finance care? Are you or your spouse retired? Will there be retirement income in addition to Social Security? Is there health insurance? Does it cover both of you? Is either of you covered by Medicare? How much is in retirement plans and can you get a lump sum withdrawal, or only monthly payments? Can you get hardship withdrawals?

If resources are insufficient, there are supplemental resources available at the national, state, and local levels. Although there are minor differences between Oregon and Virginia, it is important to know that they provide very similar and extensive services for caregivers, as your state most likely does as well. It is important to know that support for caregivers is tiered. There are national programs available for every state and caregiver; state agencies dedicated to providing services to the elderly and infirm; and many of these services are administered through county and city departments in addition to their own services.

- National
- Affordable Care Act (Obamacare)/health insurance
- Medicare
- Medicaid (administered through the state)

State Resources in Oregon[68] and Virginia[69]

In Oregon, the Area Agencies on Aging provides assistance with senior benefit programs, Social Security, Medicare, eligibility for low-income senior programs including home and community services (some states will provide part-time caregiving in the home through their home and community services program), along with:

- Caregiver training
- Case management
- Healthy aging programs
- Home-delivered meals
- Prescription drug programs
- Senior activities
- Support groups
- Transportation
- Volunteer opportunities

Virginia has the Offices for Aging Services, Dementia Services. This department focuses on dementia and provides a number of services for caregivers and the diagnosed. Major areas of services for caregivers are:

- Adult day care
- Care transitions
- Case management/care coordination

---

68 http://www.caregiverlist.com/oregon/departmentonaging.aspx
69 https://www.vda.virginia.gov/dementia.htm

- Check-ins (telephone reassurance)
- Chores
- Chronic disease self-management education (CDSME)
- Communication, information, and referral assistance (CRIA)
- Counseling services
- Disease prevention and health promotion
- Meals and nutrition services
- No wrong door (NWD) aging resources
- Ombudsmen
- Options counseling
- Personal care services
- Public guardianship
- Residential repair and renovation programs
- Respite care initiative
- Transportation

County and city available resources are outlined through the Medford Senior Center.[70] Here are some of the services offered:

- Case management
- Community-based & institutional care
- Food stamps
- Foster home licensing
- Gatekeeper program
- Information and assistance
- In-home care
- Meals
- Medical & cash assistance

---

70 http://medfordseniorcenter.org/services/medford-senior-resources/

- Medical supplies
- Protection from abuse
- Preadmission screening
- Risk intervention

This list of services offered in Fairfax County, Virginia,[71] is edited to the most common, relevant services for caregivers:

- Adult day health care
- Adult protective services
- Care management/social work; Elderlink
- Caregiver support programs and respite
- Disability rights and resources
- Food assistance (SNAP); meals on wheels
- home repair; housing
- In-home care; home care registry
- Medicaid
- Medicare—insurance counseling (VICAP)
- Memory—insight memory care
- Mental health services
- Long-term care ombudsman program
- Nursing Homes/assisted living facilities
- SeniorNavigator (public/private services)
- Speech and hearing services
- Tax relief
- Transportation

---

71 https://www.fairfaxcounty.gov/familyservices/older-adults

Talk with Family Members

It is advisable to have a family meeting when the shock of the diagnosis subsides to develop a plan of support—for finances, sharing caregiving tasks, and to devise a schedule that provides relief for you.

In many cases, this is not a pleasant conversation, as getting financial and caregiving support may be elusive. Your children have lives of their own and may not see how they can help. This may disappoint and/or make you and your spouse angry, especially true in stepfamilies. The stepchildren may be reluctant to help a caregiving stepparent, even though it is their natural father or mother who has been diagnosed. I saw this several times in support groups; stepchildren backing away from supporting the stepparent.

However, this discussion should be held, and it will alert the family that things are not going to be the same for the next three to 20 years, depending on diagnosis. Sometimes, the family will suggest that you and the diagnosed relocate closer to a son and/or daughter, move into their home, or that your adult children should move in with you.

Moving into a child's home can be a mixed blessing; the assistance and sharing of caregiving responsibilities is certainly a plus. The difficult aspect is the stress on the child of not only the care receiver and their needs, but of adapting to a multifamily environment in one home and the lack of understanding by the child/ren of how much time, stress, and effort it takes to care for someone with dementia.

Again, I recommend that you seek out a therapist to discuss moving in with your son or daughter. All of the issues that existed when they were growing up will resurface and have to be dealt with again. Either you are the guest in their house, or they are a guest in your house, and you are back in the parent–child role. This creates additional stress to an already stressful process.

CHAPTER 6: RELATIONSHIPS

Alzheimer's gradually takes away the person you know and love. As this happens, you'll mourn him or her and may experience the phases of grieving: denial, anger, guilt, sadness, and acceptance. The stages of grief don't happen neatly in order. You may move in and out of different stages as time goes on. Some common experiences in the grieving[72] process, with emphasis added to highlight the most difficult feelings, include:

- **Denial**
    - **Hoping that the person is really not ill**
    - **Expecting the person to get better**
    - **Convincing yourself that the person hasn't changed**
    - **Attempting to normalize problematic behaviors**
- Anger
    - Being frustrated with the person
    - Resenting the demands of caregiving
    - Resenting family members who cannot or will not help provide care
    - Feeling abandoned
- **Guilt**
    - **Having unrealistic expectations of yourself**, with thoughts like, "I should have done..." "I must do everything for them" or "I must visit every day"
    - **Feeling bad because you're still able to enjoy life**
    - **Negative thoughts about the person or wishing they would go away or die**
    - **Regretting things that happened in your relationship before the diagnosis**
- Sadness
    - Feeling overwhelmed by loss

---

72 https://www.alz.org/care/alzheimers-dementia-grief-loss.asp

- Crying frequently
- Withdrawing from social activities or needing to connect more often with others
- Withholding your emotions or displaying them more openly than usual
- Acceptance
  - Learning to live in the moment
  - Finding personal meaning in caring for someone who is terminally ill
  - Understanding how the grieving process affects your life
  - Appreciating the personal growth that comes from surviving loss
  - Finding your sense of humor

Not everyone goes through each stage or in this sequence. These are types of reactions or feelings that come with grieving and may be exhibited by the person or caregiver.

The Kübler-Ross Grief Cycle

Swiss psychiatrist Elisabeth Kübler-Ross first introduced her five-stage grief model in her book *On Death and Dying*. Kübler-Ross' model was based off her work with terminally ill patients and has received much criticism, mainly because people studying her model mistakenly believed this is the specific order in which people grieve and that all people go through all stages.

Kübler-Ross Grief Cycle

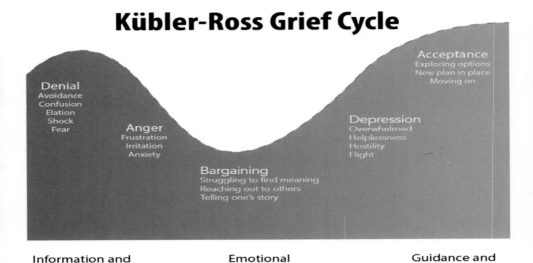

Kübler-Ross notes that these stages are not linear and some people may not experience any of them. Still, others might only undergo two or three stages rather than all five. It is now more readily known that these five stages are the most commonly observed :[73]

Denial

- You are not living in *actual reality*; you are living in a *preferable* reality.

- Interestingly, it is denial and shock that help you cope and survive the grief event.

- Denial aids in pacing feelings of grief. Instead of becoming completely overwhelmed with grief, we deny it, do not accept it, and stagger its full impact on us at one time.

- Think of it as your body's natural defense mechanism saying "Hey, there's only so much I can handle at once."

- Once the denial and shock starts to fade, the healing process begins.

- At this point, feelings that you were once suppressing are coming to the surface.

---

73 https://www.psycom.net/depression.central.grief.html

Anger

- Once you start to live in *actual* reality again and not in *preferable* reality, anger might set in.

- This is a common stage to think "Why me?" and "Life's not fair!"

- You might want to blame others for the cause of your grief or redirect your anger to close friends and family.

- You find it incomprehensible of how something like this could happen to you.

Bargaining

- You might falsely make yourself believe that you can avoid the grief through a type of negotiation: *If you change this, I'll change that.*

- You are so desperate to get your life back to how it was before the grief event, you are willing to make a major life change in an attempt toward normality.

- Guilt is a common wingman of bargaining.

Depression

- Depression is a commonly accepted form of grief.

- The world might seem too much and too overwhelming to face.

- You don't want to be around others, don't feel like talking, and experience feelings of hopelessness.

- The diagnosed might experience suicidal thoughts; "What's the point of going on?"

Acceptance

- The last stage of grief identified by Kübler-Ross is acceptance, not that "It's okay my spouse died" rather, it's "My spouse died, but I'm going to be okay."

- In this stage, your emotions may begin to stabilize. You reenter reality.

- You come to terms with the fact that the "new" reality is that (caregiver) your partner is never coming back, or that (care receiver) you are going to succumb to your illness and die soon, and you're okay with that.

Levels of Denial

There are two levels of denial. The **first level of denial** is related to the diagnosis and part of the mourning process.

Case	Care Receiver	Caregiver
Case One	**Denial**	**Denial**
Case Two	**Acceptance**	**Denial**
Case Three	**Denial**	**Acceptance**
Case Four	**Acceptance**	**Acceptance**

Case One: This is not uncommon when the diagnosis is made. Both the care receiver and caregiver go through a brief period of denial that there is a formal explanation for the "something is wrong."

Case Two: This is more common than one would think. From my experience, it usually is the care receiver that knows there is a problem with memory, but the caregiver does not accept the diagnosis or believe that it is "that bad." The caregiver will try to minimize the problem or blame it on "just getting old." I had one case in a support group where the care receiver asked to join, but the caregiver was very angry and thought that it was too early for a support group.

Case Three: This is rare, as the care receiver is most aware of the problems with memory. The acceptance by the caregiver tends to mitigate this situation.

Case Four: This is the most common case after the initial diagnosis, where the care receiver and caregiver have reconciled the situation.

The **second level of denial** was developed from my observations and from facilitating support groups. This is where the caregiver is in denial about what the care receiver's capabilities are, manifesting in the caregiver thinking that the person can stay home for an hour or more by themselves, when in reality, the care receiver is at high risk. If something should happen in the home, for instance, they leave the stove on by mistake or go outside and begin to wander, they are impaired and cannot react quickly or may not understand how to remedy a situation.

This is a result, I believe, of the caregiver thinking of how the care receiver was and not how they are now. One needs to remember that changes in behavior as a result of the disease do not have a "warning" signal. These changes can be sudden and unexpected.

Relationships

You may encounter a lack of understanding from your colleagues or boss. They may not appreciate the time it may require or the interruptions at work that may occur when you are a caregiver. This is especially true when the care receiver lives at home. Your colleagues won't realize the stress you're under from being a caregiver. It may affect your job performance. You will be taking more time off than usual or have to alter your work schedule.

There might be some resentment from colleagues because you are getting "special" treatment. Be understanding; in many cases when you take time off, they have to cover for you. The resentment may be from their feelings of covering for you and/or doing extra work to make up for the time that you are not there.

You may receive lower ratings on your job performance evaluations. Be sure to inform Human Resources and the company's employee assistance organization, if they have one, about your situation. They can help you with coping, resources, and especially if there is a job performance issue because of time off, interruptions, and/or stress.

Be sure to inform management about the diagnosis and your situation. Chances are good that someone they know is going through a similar problem. If they do not react with compassion, then loop back to HR for advice.

Building on the findings of *The Shriver Report: A Woman's Nation Takes on Alzheimer's* released in 2010, caregiving responsibilities significantly affect an individual's ability to perform job responsibilities. Among those who work(ed) while also providing care:[74]

---

74 http://www.ehstoday.com/health/how-alzheimer-s-caregiving-impacts-us-work-force

- 69% had to modify their schedules
- 32% had to take a leave of absence
- 26% changed jobs for a less-demanding role
- 20% saw their work performance suffer to the point of possible dismissal
- 69% said that caring for someone with dementia strained their family finances
- 90% characterized their caregiving as emotionally stressful

My Experience

When I told my employers about the diagnosis, they were understanding and compassionate. And when I indicated that we needed to move to Ashland, Oregon, to prepare for the placement in a memory care facility, they agreed to my telecommuting from our Ashland home. We moved two years after the diagnosis and I set up my office in the condo that we bought in a 55-plus community. I telecommuted for five years before retiring.

Family Relationships

Do not be surprised by the reaction of your immediate family. Often, members of the family deny the diagnosis and would say the parent seems "OK to me." They may minimize the issues and sometimes back away or refuse to get involved.

This is especially true when there are stepchildren. Sometimes, stepchildren complain that the caregiver is not giving the best care to their parent, but they do not assist. Or the caregiver is only supported by his/her natural children and becomes at odds with the stepchildren. Other times, stepchildren will try to step in and "replace" the caregiver; a variation on the denial in that they do not think the caregiver is providing proper care.

This is especially hard on the caregiver who is being pushed away. The reaction of other family members is one of fear that they will "come down with" dementia or Alzheimer's disease. They thus shun the care receiver, behave as though Alzheimer's is contagious, and may not assist the caregiver or do so reluctantly.

When acceptance is finally achieved, the family can become a valuable support structure in providing respite to the caregiver while they take care of other things or just gets time away.

My Experience

My daughter was very supportive; however, because of difficulties with their relationship, Nora rejected her attempts at caregiving. Anne moved from Oregon to Marin County after completing graduate school and spent six months helping me care for Nora while I was at work. But Nora would lock Anne out of the house or kick her out if she was already inside. Nora also became paranoid and verbally abusive to Anne, who decided to move back to Oregon as the situation was not helping anyone. After her move, she agreed with the placement, assisted in the hearing on spoon-feeding, and did not mind if Nora came to visit, as long as I was there.

Friends

Do not be surprised by the reaction of your friends. When in the presence of family and friends, the care receiver puts on a facade and works extremely hard at trying to appear as "normal" as possible, so your friend may say the diagnosed person seems fine. The interesting thing about this response is that it angers the caregiver because it minimizes the situation and questions the veracity of the caregiver—who is looking at a multiyear process of their partner dying.

Another caution is to watch out for "abusing" your friends' offers of help. In support groups I've heard complaints about lifelong friends not helping. Sometimes, this comes when the caregiver has leaned so much on friends that they also experience burnout or anxiety and stress. They may have the same issues that you do about caregiving.

My Experience

In the "early" days, I would take Nora with me on business trips from Ashland to the Bay Area. I would ask one of her very best friends if they would be available to care for her while I went to work. Usually, these would be just three-day trips—one travel day, one work day, and the return day to Ashland. On the third or fourth occasion, the friend that offered to help said she could not do it anymore because it was too demanding and started to interfere with her work. I accepted it, thanked her, and we are still friends.

Impact on Relationships

Below is a diagram I developed utilizing Maslow's hierarchy of needs as a base. As the disease progresses, the caregiver's life moves toward the center of the diagram. The caregiver begins to not go out as much because it becomes a major ordeal. The caregiver begins to reduce activities, does not travel, has less time for themselves, and begins to make decisions based on the impact upon the care receiver. As the disease continues to

70

progress, the caregiver enjoys fewer activities for themselves, constantly evaluates the impact of activity or decisions on the care receiver, and begins to deny their own wishes and interests. Finally, it becomes "all about the care receiver" and little or no consideration for yourself. This is when resentment, anger, and intolerance begin to appear in your behavior.

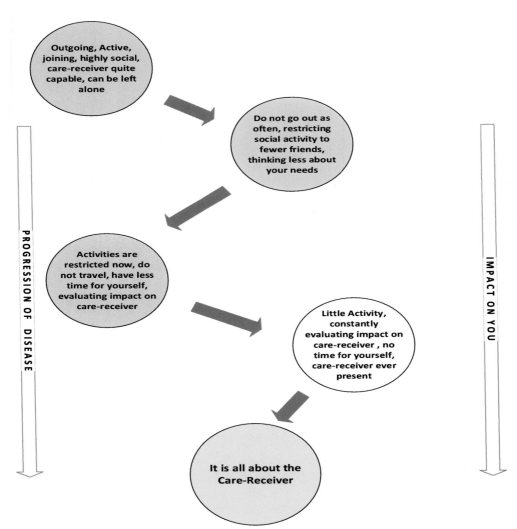

FIGURE 7: IMPACT ON RELATIONSHIPS

Support Groups

The need for joining a support group starts with the diagnosis. It is important to you and to the care receiver. There are several different types of support groups:

- Care receiver/caregiver joint meetings, basically educational; generally meet once a month
- Care receiver/caregiver joint meetings, after educational portion, split briefly into receivers and givers; generally meet once a month
- Separate meetings, one for care receivers and one for caregivers, focus is on moral support and listening; can meet weekly, bi-weekly, or once a month
- Separate meetings, one for care receivers and one for caregivers, focus is on "support" and providing therapeutic assistance and suggestions; can meet weekly, bi-weekly or once a month

My Experience

In my experience, a support group that meets only once or twice a month is less effective in all-around *support* of the caregiver; these are more effective for educational support.

My recommendation is to find a *weekly* support group that has separate meetings, one for caregivers and one for care receivers. I found that meeting weekly enables the caregiver to voice their current and most troublesome concerns. In a monthly meeting, the concerns of the first week are lost or not discussed by the time the monthly meeting comes around. However, the concern in week one is still vitally important. Meeting weekly provides more support and helps the care receiver, as well. The same problem, even more so, is present for the care receiver. They would not remember what troubled them in week one when it was week four.

Nora voiced major concerns about two things: One was *You do not know what I am going through. You cannot understand what it is like.* And two, *I am all alone.* The care receiver support group provided help on both of these concerns. She was with others who were going through the same thing she was and "understood" how it felt. Secondly, she saw that she was *not* alone; the others around the table were also diagnosed. This really mattered to Nora and it provided comfort. When she would say in the group "Bill is always bossing me around, telling me what to do and what not to do." The others in her group would say "Yeah, that makes me so mad when they boss me around," and she felt validated.

In the caregiving group, someone would say, "I just wish they would die." Others would say, "I have thought that too." It was normal to feel that way—it is hard being a caregiver.

Examples of Support Group Sponsors (Ashland, Oregon)

Alzheimer's Association of Jackson County [75]

Home Instead Senior Care (joint meeting type of group)
Second and fourth Wednesday of the month from 3:30 to 5 p.m.
81 Freeman Court
Central Point, OR 97502

Westminster Presbyterian Church (joint meeting type of group)
Third Thursday of the month from 2 to 3:30 p.m.
2000 Oakwood Drive
Medford, OR 97504

Ashland Senior Center (joint meeting type of group)
(cosponsored by Ashland Parks and Recreation)
Third Wednesday of the month from 5:30 to 7 p.m.
1699 Homes Ave.
Ashland, OR 97520

State, county and/or city senior services

Retirement residential centers
- Rogue Valley Manor
- Mountain Meadows

Memory care facilities
- Table Rock Memory Care (previously Fern Gardens), Medford
- Farmington, Medford
- Valley View, Ashland

Not-for-profit senior organizations
- AARP

Private health consultants
- Power of the Heart: Dementia Care Education and Behavior Coaching! (Marya Kain)

---

75 https://www.alz.org/oregon/in_my_community_20728.asp#Jackson

- Anam Cara Center for Learning and Care, The Memory Care Project (Elizabeth V. Hallett Consulting)

Examples of Support Group Sponsors (Fairfax, Virginia)

Alzheimer's Association for Fairfax County[76]

Aldersgate United Methodist Church
1301 Collingwood Road
Alexandria, VA 22308
Second Thursday of the month from 7:30–9pm.
RSVP Required: Joan Sutton (202) 285-6486

Goodwin House
4800 Fillmore Avenue
Alexandria, VA 22311
Second Saturday of the month at 10:30 a.m.
RSVP Required: Karen Profitt (508) 400-1703

Tysons-Pimmit Library Virtual via Zoom
7584 Leesburg Pike
Falls Church, VA 22043
Fourth Tuesday of the month at 7 p.m.
RSVP Required: Rebecca Greene, rfgreene2@yahoo.com (703) 587-4301; co-facilitator Colleen Duewel

Historic Silas Burke House
9617 Burke Lake Road
Burke, VA 22015
Fourth Sunday of the month at 2 p.m.
RSVP Required: Phyllis Humphrey, humphreypm@aol.com

Alexandria Support Group
Virtual support group
3rd Sunday at 2:00 p.m.
Lori Woelfel, bankingonamemory@gmail.com; co-facilitator Shawn Ulrick

---

76 https://www.alz.org/getattachment/nca/Helping_You/Support_Groups/Support-Groups-5_27_2021_NoVA.pdf

It's a necessity that at least the caregiver goes to a support group. From my experience and the feedback from support groups that I have facilitated, the benefits of joining a support group are overwhelming.

Therapy

You will need to learn coping skills and how to take care of yourself in this long mourning process. Find a nonjudgmental person to talk with about coping with the loss of companionship and physical contact or sex. Remember Maslow's hierarchy of needs.

For adult children who are caregivers to their parents, I find this vitally important for several reasons. All of the issues that the son or daughter had while growing up come back again with a twist: The parent becomes the child and the child becomes the parent. Dormant or repressed emotions are revisited and may become difficult to manage.

Sometimes the person with dementia reacts with "Who are you to tell me what to do?" The child may become intolerant of the behaviors the person with dementia exhibits, especially if they become belligerent or hostile. A therapist will help the child cope with these issues.

When the person with dementia enters the later stages of the disease and hospice is involved, a therapist can be a great help to the caregiver in coping with the impending death, the mourning process, and in many cases, the isolation.

My Experience

We each had a therapist in Northern California shortly after the diagnosis. When we arrived in Ashland, I located a therapist as did Nora. She went to a different therapist to deal with her issues and coping with the diagnosis but eventually ceased to benefit because of the progression of the disease.

My therapist helped me in many ways. A couple stand out:

- He kept reminding me that Nora, the person I married, was no longer there (the second level of denial)
- He made me feel comfortable about placing her and dealing with the reality that she is not "coming back"
- He helped me deal with the process of placing Nora in a memory care facility and dealing with my emotions about it

- After working *with* me on placement, he worked *on* me to deal with my social isolation and lack of companionship and physical contact.
- He encouraged me to go on dates, and if necessary, join match.com—he assured me that it was all right and appropriate.
- Socializing was neither easy nor totally welcome because of guilt.

The upshot is that I met Marilyn and we "dated" for five years before marrying in July 2018. She understood and accepted the situation when we met and while we dated.

CHAPTER 7: Tough Decisions

Because of the disease and its progression, you will be required to make tough decisions for the care receiver, even though you think they are capable of participating or of consensus on these decisions. Throughout our relationships with the (care receiver) partner or parent, we have automatically incorporated their input capabilities into important matters, such as where to live, if we need a new car, if we should continue to work, to entertain, etc.

Alzheimer's and dementia now make simple activities or tasks a major decision point in the relationship. One needs to take into account that the care receiver is less likely to be rational about some of these major issues; they depend on familiarity and routine for well-being, so any major change is met with a negative response. Deciding to sell our second car because only one of us should be driving was met with a firm, "No! I need it."

Remember, **you** must make the decision and disregard the wishes of the care receiver. They are not rational about these issues because of the disease. It has robbed them of perspective and objectivity. Below are many of the major issues that will require you to make such a decision.

Driving

Driving is one of the most contentious issues between the care receiver and the caregiver. From teenager to mature adult, driving is a sign of independence, self-sustenance, and identity for men as well as women.

However, women generally do not have same kind of attachment to cars as men. In support groups, driving was the most difficult issue discussed because, one, wanting to avoid conflict, and two, the second level of denial.

Rarely discussed is the avoidance of conflict. In most cases, it engenders an argument, leading right into the second level of denial by convincing themselves that they are really fine to drive. *When I am with them their driving does seem fine—although sometimes I have to help them find their way and warn them of traffic situations.*

Liability is one of the best rationales for not letting one drive when they have a formal diagnosis of dementia or Alzheimer's. In the support groups, I asked *What is the likelihood that a driving accident, where you would go to court or need a lawyer, would be decided in your favor after it came out that the driver had Alzheimer's disease?* I also mention that they should contact their insurance company and let them know that a formal diagnosis has been made and ask what the consequences are for the caregiver.

Most states require that the diagnosing doctor contacts the department of motor vehicles when a diagnosis of Alzheimer's or dementia is made. The DMV is supposed to make a determination of if and when the person should be retested and whether it would be a written and/or driving test. I have found the DMV generally does not follow up on these notifications unless you ask them to.

There is one way of interjecting a third party (such as the DMV) into this touchy subject; the occupational therapist that specializes in driving tests for impaired drivers. They are generally associated with a hospital. The American Occupational Therapy Association describes the role of the driving therapist as follows:[77]

Occupational therapy practitioners with specialized training in driver rehabilitation may administer comprehensive driving evaluations. This type of driving evaluation typically includes two parts: one part in an office or clinic, the second part behind the wheel of a car. The purpose of the evaluation in the office or clinic is to examine the physical, visual, and mental abilities required for safe driving. This would include:

- Reaction time, needed for stopping fast enough to avoid a crash;
- Basic visual acuity, or sharpness of vision; and
- Decision-making, judgment, and planning (i.e., needed for making left turns).

The behind-the-wheel or on-road part of the evaluation takes place in a vehicle equipped with safety equipment such as an instructor's brake. The on-road evaluation identifies an older driver's strengths and weaknesses and ways to keep driving safely. If necessary, the evaluation may use adaptive equipment.

In Medford, Oregon, The Providence Driving Assessment[78] can help determine if it is safe for someone to continue driving. An occupational therapist works with each client to determine driver safety. The assessment includes:

- Review of the client's driving history
- Visual screening

---

77 https://www.aota.org/Practice/Productive-Aging/Driving/Clients/Evaluate/Eval-by-OT.aspx
78 https://oregon.providence.org/our-services/d/driver-assessment/

- Physical screening to measure range of motion, strength, and coordination
- Cognitive and perceptual screening
- Evaluation of functional mobility
- An on-the-road driving test is not part of the evaluation. This assessment measures a person's ability to drive safely. It can ease concerns about drivers who experience health-related incidents or declining health but who wish to continue driving.
- In Alexandria, Virginia, Rachel Feinstein, OTR/L, CDRS is an outpatient occupational therapist.[79] She is associated with Inova Mount Vernon Hospital and is currently only treating the following conditions:
  - Stroke/CVA, brain injury, concussion, spinal cord injury, amputations, neuropathy, Parkinson's, multiple sclerosis, Guillain barre syndrome, **dementia, Alzheimer's,** autism, and Asperger's (driving simulator—3W restriction not required) (emphasis added)

Here are some possible ways to stop people with Alzheimer's disease from driving:[80]
- Try talking about your concerns with the person
- Take him or her to get a driving test
- Ask the doctor to tell him or her to stop driving; the doctor can write, "Do not drive" on a prescription pad, and you can show this to the person
- Move to another state; I did
- **Hide the car keys, move the car, take out the distributor cap, or disconnect the battery** [emphasis added]

Hiding the keys: When asked, you can say *You had them last, I do not know where they are, let's look for them* (but not find them). However, this does not have a high success rate. (This is a last resort when all else fails.)

Talk with the care receiver about driving as part of the discussions after diagnosis. Try to set up criteria for when to stop driving, such as, losing your way home, a close call, or minor accident. This is difficult, because when the driver crosses that criteria, it is already too late.

You can have one of the children talk with the care receiver and indicate that it is time to stop driving. This does not make *you* the bad guy, and sometimes it is more acceptable to the care receiver.

---

79 2501 Parker's Lane, Alexandria, VA 22306. Voice: 703-664-7190 Fax:703-664-7423. feinsteinr@gmail.com
80 https://www.nia.nih.gov/health/driving-safety-and-alzheimers-disease

You can also call the DMV anonymously to report a driver who has been diagnosed and should be retested or reexamined.

You can elicit the help of family members to discuss the issue and help you enforce *your* decision that the care receiver should not be driving. The problem with family members is that they do not want to be the one that tells the person they should not be driving.

The main reason the person with dementia should not be driving is that the disease impairs the ability to make split-second decisions in an unpredictable situation. This could lead to someone being hurt or killed because the impaired driver could not react in time. You don't want to be answering that why they were still allowed to drive was because you wanted to avoid an argument.

My Experience

When I was 16 and got my first car, I saw it as a symbol of adulthood, independence, and freedom of movement. Many drivers do. It was important to Nora and was also a sign of independence and freedom. With Nora's agreement (and that of her therapist), I had an occupational therapist give Nora a driving test within a year of diagnosis. The therapist had Nora drive our car around our area, then took her to San Francisco and UCSF Medical School where she had her doctor's appointments—15 to 20 miles from where we lived—which included driving across the Golden Gate Bridge. It was reported that she was okay around where we lived but had difficulties when they went to UCSF. The recommendation was that she could drive nearby, but not outside of our county.

I was disappointed in the recommendation because I thought she shouldn't be driving at all, but I acquiesced. We moved to Ashland in July 2011 and she continued to drive locally, until one day she went to Safeway, a mile or so from the house. About an hour later, she called me, hysterical, saying she could not find her way home. This was especially frightening because I had no way to know where she was and she was not capable of telling me where she was. Finally, she stumbled her way home. This was less than six months after we moved.

I reiterated that she needed to go to the DMV and get an Oregon driver's license. I was pretty sure that she would not pass the written test; hence, problem solved—no driver's license and I was not the bad guy. A professional caregiver who came during the week while I telecommuted took her to the DMV where she failed the written test and got an ID card instead. She stopped driving. I was lucky—the DMV became the bad guy and told her not to drive. Many in the support group are not so lucky. But a retest at the DMV is an option.

Removing Favorite Items

When and how do you remove guns, shop tools, and other items that are potentially unsafe? These may be major components of the care receiver's hobbies and activities.

This too can be difficult; however, it is not as traumatic as driving. Guns seem to be the hardest, as they hold a special place for the receiver. Guns usually apply more to men who have been diagnosed than to women. The reason for owning a gun is protection, hunting, or sport. It is the protection aspect that usually makes care receivers most upset about giving up their guns; they feel exposed, vulnerable, and unsafe as the disease progresses. The gun makes them feel safer and more secure.

Guns are especially dangerous because as the disease progresses, the care receiver may become hostile, suffer from hallucinations, and even become violent or physically abusive.[81] One woman in a support group said that she took the guns and sold them without telling the receiver. When he asked, she said that she did not know where he put them. Another caregiver was too afraid to take the guns away, so we recommended that when he was out, to hide the guns or give them to their children for safekeeping. When he asked about them, she also indicated that she did not know what he did with his guns since he was the last to take them out.

Even electric or power tools are unsafe for the care receiver. Remember, the disease impairs the ability to make decisions, especially split-second decisions. Power tools present a problem if they are an integral part of the care receiver's persona and working with them is a gratifying, high self-esteem activity, especially if they are very skilled with the tools.

You really have to fight the second level of denial to keep them from using the tools as the disease progresses. Their hobbies bring such joy to them that you feel bad when you

---

81 https://www.cnn.com/2018/06/27/health/guns-dementia-partner/index.html "A four-month Kaiser Health News investigation has uncovered dozens of cases across the US in which people with dementia used guns to kill or injure themselves or others. From news reports, court records, hospital data and public death records, KHN found 15 homicides and more than 60 suicides since 2012, although there are likely many more. The shooters often **acted during bouts of confusion, paranoia, delusion or aggression** [emphasis added]—common symptoms of dementia. They killed people closest to them—their caretaker, wife, son, or daughter. They shot at people they happened to encounter—a mailman, a police officer, a train conductor. At least four men with dementia who brandished guns were fatally shot by police. In cases where charges were brought, many assailants were deemed incompetent to stand trial. Many killed themselves. Among men in the US, the suicide rate is highest among those 65 and older; firearms are the most common method according to the Centers for Disease Control and Prevention. These statistics do not begin to tally incidents in which a person with dementia waves a gun at an unsuspecting neighbor or a terrified home health aide." Also see http://mailtribune.com/news/top-stories/unlocked-and-loaded-the-deadly-intersection-between-dementia-and-guns

try to discourage use. Their attitude is that they can do it or can make a certain change or repair, when the reality is, they cannot.

One person took all the power cords away and told the care receiver that the tools were broken and could not be used. She did not explain to him why the power tools did not work. This is an extreme example, but she indicated that he would not listen to her.

Taking other things away may not be as difficult as they go into disuse as the disease progresses and the care receiver loses interest or the capability to use them. Another woman sold an antique car over the care receiver's objections.

Remember, these are *tough* decisions you have to make as this disease progresses. These are things to look at and decide if the receiver should be using or performing these activities. It is another reason for having a trust and putting all of these items in it so that you can dispose of them without the care receiver's consent.

Selling these items may provide conflict in the house, as they will say no when asked if you can get rid of them. But the main thing to remember is that they are not rational although they appear and talk as though they are—reinforcing the second level of denial.

They enter what I call the "elder terrible twos." Everything that you want to remove, sell, and/or change will generally be met with a No! by the care receiver. Again, routine, familiarity, and the caregiver are the lynchpins of stability and normalcy. When we caregivers want to make a major change in their routine or their surroundings, it will be met with negativism and sometimes hostility or an argument.

That is why I say the decision is made by *you* and not by the care receiver, nor necessarily with the care receiver's consent. Conflict may not be avoided. One member of a support group told the group that his wife would get really mad and go into the bedroom and *slam* the door. About 15 minutes later, she would come out and interact as though nothing had happened. In other words, they will not be angry forever nor, hopefully, for long. A small, positive side effect of the disease.

Entertaining

As the disease progresses, the care receiver in a formal or large gathering will:

- Isolate/sit by themselves
- Withdraw from the main group or activity
- Stop talking and not really be listening

82

The issue is that these gatherings or entertaining a number of people at once is overwhelming their capabilities to follow conversations. Joining in and making relevant comments is impaired because they respond slower than "normal" people, making their comments seem out of place. They know they are having difficulty and may result in withdrawing from the conversation, or even from the room. It is also very tiring; they try to so hard to be "ordinary" and join in. It can be exhausting.

A caregiver should recognize and understand these issues and not place the person in such situations, even events like Thanksgiving or a Christmas, where there might be 10 or 20 people, It is very uncomfortable and keeps reminding them that they are having major difficulties.

The caregiver also does not have a good time because they are constantly monitoring their partner, and may become stressed at the care receiver's withdrawal. Or, the caregiver may become embarrassed by the comments or actions of the care receiver.

This also applies to sporting events, concerts, conventions, and so forth. These gatherings are especially difficult as they are in large, unfamiliar venues, very confusing, with lots of people moving around and action that is not specifically directed at the care receiver. It is difficult for them to follow, be engaged, or understand what is going on. So, they will become angry and frustrated or want to retreat to an out-of-the-way place. Some might even get lost in the crowd and become frightened because they do not know where you are.

Most importantly, you will not have a good time; you will be consumed with how your partner/spouse/parent is doing and concentrating on making it a good time for them. Your focus will be on care receiver and not the event, which will be frustrating to you as well.

When should you start to reduce entertaining friends or going to events?

My Experience

I found that I just naturally reduced our entertaining as the disease progressed. Nora would lose interest in the conversation around the dinner table, just get up and go sit in the living room, or disengage from the group. The main reasons were that she found it very hard to follow the conversation, to join in and make appropriate comments, or the topics moved too fast for her. I found the getting up and going into the living room alone the hardest to take as it always stopped the conversation and elicited a comment about her illness, generally shortening the evening. So, I just stopped asking people over for dinner, drinks, or visits.

I also found myself restricting what events we went to. I declined invitations because Nora would have a hard time. I would refuse invitations to dinner parties if there were going to be more than four other people. She would sometimes become so frustrated that she would become hostile or rude. She would also be very tired and melancholy afterward.

Leaving the Person Home Alone

When is it not appropriate to leave the receiver home alone? This is a classic decision where the second level of denial really comes into play. The caregiver thinks that the care receiver is quite capable of staying home alone, because they just sit around or watch TV anyway; they do not go outside on their own. They tell you they will be fine and you have a white board telling them where you are going and when you will be home.

None of the above is enough. As mentioned earlier, the progression of the disease and behaviors are unpredictable. One caregiver went downstairs to exercise while the care receiver was upstairs reading. When he finished, she was nowhere to be found. She had put on her coat and went outside to go to church (on a weekday) and started walking. He had no warning signs that she was going to start wandering. She was found two miles from the house walking in the wrong direction. A neighbor saw her and drove her home. The moral here is there was no warning or indication that she would wander, it just happened. Just as leaving the stove on or not being able to find their way home from a walk, all are behaviors that could not have been predicted.

Also, if there is an emergency, such as a fall, or a fire, or an earthquake, the receiver may not know how to deal with the situation or how to get help. Or, more likely, someone comes to the door (a salesperson, charity, delivery person, a scam artist, *et al.*), and the care receiver may invite them into the house, give them money, or both.

Some think that leaving your phone number will suffice; however, many times the care receiver will not know how to operate a phone or may not remember information is on the white board. If they do not know where you are or cannot see you, they may panic.

In summary, remember that as the disease progresses, the care receiver becomes less rational and cannot make good decisions.

My Experience

I tried to not leave Nora home alone but with a neighbor, caregiver, or friend. She did not like this, but it gave me peace of mind. In one group, a person told us that she got so fed up with the situation and stress that she just left the care receiver, who was in a wheelchair, and went to a movie. If there had been an emergency, the person may not have been able to get out of the house or even to the door.

In our small, 900 square foot condo, she would come into the bedroom/office and say "Oh, there you are." She needed the reassurance of the visual sighting to understand that I was there. Otherwise, she thought I was not.

You have to really fight the second level of denial. You think they are more capable and rational than they really are and want to get out, run an errand, meet friends, or go to an event and you convince yourself that they are quite capable of staying by themselves for an hour or two.

In support groups, I would challenge the group to evaluate their situation by looking at their anxiety level when getting home. As they get closer, park the car, go up to the door— does anxiety increase? I suspect it does. You are thinking, *What am I going to find? Are they home or did they wander? Are they where I left them or have they fallen, injured themselves? Is everything okay? Is the stove off?* When you enter, you find all is well, and your anxiety dissipates almost immediately, it means they should not stay at home alone, because it is not good for *you*! You will be distracted and anxious at your luncheon, wondering if they are "behaving" themselves.

It is completely different if you have someone there while you are gone. You know they are okay and any emergency will be taken care of and any surprise will be handled by the person staying with the care receiver. When you are coming home, parking the car, going to the door, and coming inside there is little or no anxiety on your part, because someone is there with the care receiver. It lowers your stress! And the other side of the coin is it lowers the stress of the care receiver as well. Someone is there for them, they feel safer.

Travel

When is it not appropriate for them to travel, alone or with you? This is another tough decision, as the travel may be to family or favorite relatives. However, to me, traveling is one of the more stressful activities that a caregiver engages in, because the threat of losing track of the person in a totally strange place is very high. This is especially true with air travel and going through security. A simple task like going to the restroom can become a harrowing experience. During one group session, a co-facilitator described such an experience in an airport. His wife wanted to go to the bathroom and so he stood outside the entrance waiting for her. When she seemed to be taking longer than expected he began to look around to see if he missed her coming out of the bathroom. He discovered that there was another exit down the hall; lucky for him, he spotted her walking away. The suggestion was to use a "family" bathroom and go in with the person in the future so they do not get lost; whether it is you who needs to go or the other person.

It is not uncommon to get separated in an airport, whether at security, on the way to the gate, at the boarding gate, perusing a newsstand, at the luggage carousel, etc. Getting separated can be a frightening experience for both of you.

If you are going to travel, tell the desk attendant that the person with you has dementia/Alzheimer's so they can be a resource if the caregiver needs help.

My Experience

I want to reduce my stress and not have trips turn into nightmares. When I felt uncomfortable about leaving my spouse home alone, I figured it was time to stop traveling. It is better to ask people to come to your place.

I drove to the Bay Area on a business trip one time and brought Nora. I made arrangements to have one of her friends spend the day with her while I was at work. When I returned in the late afternoon, Nora was just sitting on the couch in the lobby of the motel where we were staying. Fortunately, I had told the desk clerk that Nora had Alzheimer's, so she watched out for her. She told me that Nora just sat there for about an hour. Nora did not remember what room she was staying in or even where it was. Thankfully, the desk clerk did not think it was wise to take Nora to her room and just leave her there.

The friend that provided caregiving for Nora had known her for 30 years. She would take Nora shopping or to lunch or to a museum. On this trip, the friend told me that it was not a good idea to bring her with me again. She was not good company, needed to be monitored constantly, and it was not easy for her. I thanked her profusely for her frankness and did not take Nora with me again. We have to be aware of the stress that friends experience and not burn them out on caregiving. If it is stressful for *you* to be a caregiver, it is *very* stressful for friends/family to be caregivers.

NOTE: The goal of these tough decisions is to *lower* your stress! When you let the care receiver drive when they shouldn't, it increases your stress. When you take them to large gatherings or dinner parties, it increases your stress. When you travel with them—especially air travel—it increases your stress. These are tough decisions but should be made to lower your stress and keep them safe. Avoiding a conflict will not lower your stress.

Moving

At some point during your partner's struggle with Alzheimer's or dementia, you may have to move. You may want to downsize from a big house or remote neighborhood. Or, you have to move to a cheaper environment or assisted living community. Or, maybe a professional caregiver will move into your home.

Moving has its own issues and stress. Selling what is familiar and moving to a new community that is totally unfamiliar may confuse the care receiver. They will not know where the bathroom is, how the kitchen is organized, where their bedroom may be. There will be unfamiliar neighbors to meet and a new neighborhood to navigate. It may produce tension between the caregiver and the care receiver: "Why did we have to move? I do not like it here."

Moving may not be a choice but a necessity to reduce expenses to continue to pay for outside caregivers. Remember, *it is your decision*, not a joint decision. You may discuss it; however, the care receiver will probably disagree when asked. They are not rational nor can fully understand the situation.

The moving experience will cause anxiety and possibly anger in the care receiver. It is best to not discuss the actual move activities and have the care receiver out the house when packing or when the movers come. The care receiver will not fully understand what is happening and their presence may make the move more difficult. Their lack of understanding will raise your already high stress level.

My Experience

When we moved to Ashland two years after diagnosis, I kept Nora occupied with the help of friends. I choose Ashland because it was familiar to her—we had been going to Oregon Shakespeare Festival plays for 25 years. With Ashland familiar to her, it avoided a lot of confusion and angst and she knew her way around downtown. In moving to a 55-plus community, many friendly and understanding residents offered to help.

Sex (Yes, Sex and Intimacy)[82]

There will be changes in intimacy and sexuality. Alzheimer's disease can cause changes in both the person with the disease and the caregiver. The person with Alzheimer's may be stressed by the changes in his or her memory and behaviors. Fear, worry, depression,

---

82 https://www.nia.nih.gov/health/changes-intimacy-and-sexuality-alzheimers-disease

87

anger, and low self-esteem are common. They may become dependent and cling to you. He or she may not remember your life together or your feelings toward one another. The person may even think they've fallen in love with someone else.

You, the caregiver, may pull away from the person emotionally and physically. You may resent the demands of caregiving. You also may feel frustrated by the person's constant forgetfulness, repeated questions, and other behaviors. Most caregivers learn how to cope with these challenges, but it takes time. Some learn to live with the illness and find new meaning in their relationship with the person who has the disease.

Most people with Alzheimer's need to feel that someone loves and cares about them. They also need to spend time with other people. Your efforts to take care of these needs can help them feel happy and safe. It's important to reassure the person that:

- You love him or her
- Others also care about them
- You will keep them safe

The following tips may help you cope with your own needs:

- Talk with a doctor, social worker, or clergy member about these changes
- Talk about your concerns in a support group
- Think more about the positive parts of the relationship

Either spouse/partner may lose interest in having sex. This change can make the other feel lonely or frustrated. You may feel that:

- It's not okay to have sex with someone who has Alzheimer's
- The person with Alzheimer's seems like a stranger
- The person with Alzheimer's seems to forget that the spouse/partner is even there or how to make love

A person with Alzheimer's disease may have *side effects from medications* that affect their sexual interest as well as *memory loss, changes in the brain,* or *depression* that affect their interest in sex. Here are some tips for coping with changes in sexuality:

- Explore new ways of spending time together
- Focus on other ways to show affection, such as snuggling or holding hands
- Try other nonsexual forms of touching, such as massage, hugging, and dancing
- Consider other ways to meet your sexual needs; some caregivers report that they masturbate

There may be also the opposite effect—hypersexuality. Some people with Alzheimer's disease are overly interested in sex; they may masturbate a lot or try to seduce others. These behaviors are symptoms of the disease and don't always mean that the person wants to have sex. To cope with hypersexuality:

- Try giving the person more attention and reassurance
- You might gently touch, hug, or use other kinds of affection to meet his or her emotional needs
- Some people with this problem need medicine to control their behaviors; t*alk to a doctor* about what steps to take

Again, a therapist will be of great value in helping to deal with this very intimate and personal issue.

My Experience

Shortly after Nora was diagnosed, there were changes in her physically. Her vagina became thin and experienced a tear, stopping all intercourse. She also showed no interest in sex (even though several times men at the memory care center tried to be intimate with her). This started in 2010. I used masturbation as a substitute.

When I placed her in January 2013, I started to date a few months later, in part to have physical companionship. My therapist worked with me on how to date and have relationships. I sought out dinners with others. We were rebuilding and re-socializing me.

In Chapter 4, the diagram showed how our life moved from enriching ourselves to where it was all about the care receiver. Any decision, action, or activity was first evaluated as to the impact on the care receiver before determining what was good for us, the caregiver. In many cases, the decision, action, or activity was modified to accommodate the care receiver's needs.

The therapist worked with me to reverse the flow and reintegrate me into a social life that was independent of Nora. She was being well taken care of in the memory care center; I did not have to worry about her needs. The therapist kept telling me that the Nora I married was gone. She was not coming home.

My needs for socialization and self-actualization were not being met. The therapist worked with me to assuage the guilt and difficulties in reengaging socially and in intimacy.

CHAPTER 8: ETHICAL DECISIONS

There are ethical decisions you will face as a result of the advance directive and the progression of the disease, relating to the life and death of the care receiver.

- Do I faithfully implement the advance directive of the care receiver?
- Do I permit assisted feeding of the care receiver when they can no longer feed themselves?
- Do I advocate for VSED (voluntarily stopping eating and drinking)[83] for the care receiver?
- Do I stop life-prolonging medications (such as statins, Aricept, etc.,) when they are placed in a memory care facility or enter middle or late stages of the disease?
- Do I keep detrimental foods, snacks, or candies from diabetics or others with dietary restrictions when they enter later stages of the disease?
- Do I "violate" my vows by placing them into a memory care facility?
- Do I "date" while they are in a memory care facility?

What do I mean when I say "faithfully implement the advance directive" in the first question? If you have been designated as agent for the care receiver, you must fully understand the wishes of the care receiver when it comes the advance directive. I have included Nora's advance directive as an example. It does not matter if I disagree with her choices or wishes, as her agent, I must speak for her and her wishes. If you cannot speak for the care receiver and their wishes because of ethical conflicts with your own beliefs and moral code, then you **must not** be their agent. It will be a violation of the advance directive.

For example, if a care receiver does not want to have tube feeding, but their spouse, their agent, believes in tube feeding, the spouse/agent would have to not let the medical staff provide tube feeding, even though the agent believes in it and would want care receiver to live as long as possible.

---

83 https://compassionandchoices.org/end-of-life-planning/learn/vsed/

My Experience

Nora indicated in her advance directive that she did not choose to prolong life. This guided my voicing of Nora's wishes when it came to the above ethical issues and decisions. I placed her so that she would get better care than I could provide. The placement also enabled me to better manage her care, especially when it comes to the following issues:

- To not spoon-feed her. I gave the instructions to offer her food, however, if she could not feed herself or did not eat; that met her advance directive.

- To not provide her statins (anti-cholesterol) and Aricept (slows the pace of Alzheimer's disease), medications that I determined extended her life. I continued her thyroid medicine as I determined this was a comfort medicine, not one to prolong life.

I was able to convey these and other wishes Nora had to the staff of the memory care facility, to the doctor who visited the memory care center weekly, and to hospice. They supported her wishes.

I did notice that after two rounds of hospice, the facility was assisting in feeding Nora rather than letting her have finger food. This came about because an ombudsman requested that Nora be provided with "… three nutritious meals, and if she is unable to feed herself, provide assistance in feeding." She regained some weight and was dropped from hospice.

I felt this was against Nora's wishes and advance directive instructions. I went to my lawyer and we engaged in a court hearing to request that they stop spoon-feeding her. The upshot was that we were confronted with an Oregon administrative rule that required institutions like the memory care center to provide three meals and assist in feeding if the person was unable to do so. The judge completely concurred with the understanding that Nora did not want to be spoon-fed, but did not overturn the administrative rule, so we lost. The facility continued to spoon-feed her. This extended her life, precisely against her advance directive, and she experienced the full gamut of Alzheimer's disease, a process that took 15 months from the court's decision.

It was at that time that I learned of VSED. An attorney from Minneapolis contacted me and asked if it was possible to use Nora as an example of the need for VSED. He was going to give a talk at a conference for lawyers and doctors in Seattle. I said yes.

The important point here is that I followed Nora's advance directive and did **not** feel any remorse or guilt in going to court to challenge the ombudsman and the Oregon administrative rule.

The hearing became a national *cause célèbre*. Articles appeared in *USA Today*, the *Washington Post* and the *Medford Tribune* about the hearing and spoon-feeding. It became a topic of discussion for conferences on medical ethics and the legal system. We are still lobbying the State Legislature of Oregon to allow the advance directive to supersede the administrative rule when in conflict.

I also discussed with hospice Nora's wishes in the advanced directive concerning pain, in which she stated "… I direct that treatment for the alleviation of pain and discomfort be provided at all times, even if it hastens my death."

I noticed that Nora was restless and exhibited what I took to be discomfort and pain, even though she could not verbally communicate it. I worked with hospice to provide morphine more frequently than was scheduled. I even suggested that they provided larger doses than what would be considered safe, but they refused.

I have included Nora's advance directive to highlight the areas that can present ethical issues to the caregiver.

ADVANCE HEALTH CARE DIRECTIVE
(California Probate Code Section 4701)
Explanation

You have the right to give instructions about your own health care. You also have the right to name someone else to make health care decisions for you. This form lets you do either or both of these things. It also lets you express your wishes regarding donation of organs and the designation of your primary physician. If you use this form, you may complete or modify all or any part of it. You are free to use a different form.

Part 1 of this form is a power of attorney for health care. Part 1 lets you name another individual as agent to make health care decisions for you if you become incapable of making your own decisions or if you want someone else to make those decisions for you now even though you are still capable. You may also name an alternate agent to act for you if your first choice is not willing, able, or reasonably available to make decisions for you. (Your agent may not be an operator or employee of a community care facility or a residential care facility where you are receiving care, or your supervising health care provider or employee of the health care institution where you are receiving care, unless your agent is related to you or is a coworker.) Unless the form you sign limits the authority of your agent, your agent may make all health care decisions for you. This form has a place for you to limit the authority of your agent. You need not limit the authority of your agent if you wish to rely on your agent for all health care decisions that may have to be made. If you choose not to limit the authority of your agent, your agent will have the right to:

    (a) Consent or refuse consent to any care, treatment, service, or procedure to maintain, diagnose, or otherwise affect a physical or mental condition.

    (b) Select or discharge health care providers and institutions.

    (c) Approve or disapprove diagnostic tests, surgical procedures, and programs of medication.

    (d) Direct the provision, withholding, or withdrawal of artificial nutrition and hydration and all other forms of health care, including cardiopulmonary resuscitation.

    (e) Make anatomical gifts, authorize an autopsy, and direct disposition of remains.

Part 2 of this form lets you give specific instructions about any aspect of your health care, whether or not you appoint an agent. Choices are provided for you to express your wishes regarding the provision, withholding, or withdrawal of treatment to keep you alive, as well as the provision of pain relief. Space is also provided for you to add to the choices you have made or for you to write out any additional wishes. If you are satisfied to allow your agent to determine what is best for you in making end-of-life decisions, you need not fill out Part 2 of this form.

Exhibit "A" to this form lets you express an intention to donate your bodily organs and tissues following your death.

After completing this form, sign and date the form at the end and have your signature notarized. You may wish to give a copy of the signed and completed form to your physician, to any other health care providers you may have, to any health care institution at which you are receiving care, and to any health care agents you have named. You should talk to the person you have named as agent to be sure he or she is willing to serve.

1.

PART I: POWER OF ATTORNEY FOR HEALTH CARE

I revoke all prior advance health care directives and durable powers of attorney for health care signed by me. This document shall not be affected by my subsequent incapacity. I am not a patient in a skilled nursing facility, and I am not a conservatee.

1.1 NAME AND ADDRESS OF PRINCIPAL.   My name and address are:

Nora R. Harris, ▮▮▮▮▮▮▮▮▮ Novato, CA 94949

1.2 DESIGNATION OF AGENTS.

     a. PRIMARY AGENT. I designate the following individual as my agent to make health care decisions for me:

William L. Harris, ▮▮▮▮▮▮▮▮▮ Novato, CA 94949

     b. FIRST ALTERNATE AGENT. If I revoke my agent's authority or if my agent is not willing, able or reasonably available to make a health care decision for me, I designate as my first alternate agent:

Anne G. Harris, ▮▮▮▮▮▮▮▮▮, Eugene, OR 97401

     c. SECOND ALTERNATE AGENT. If I revoke the authority of my agent and first alternate agent or if neither is willing, able, or reasonably available to make a health care decision for me, I designate as my second alternate agent:

Margery Harris, ▮▮▮▮▮▮▮▮▮ Shell Beach, CA 93449

1.3 AGENT'S AUTHORITY.   Unless I otherwise specify in Exhibit "A", my agent is authorized to make all health care decisions for me, including decisions to provide, withhold, or withdraw artificial nutrition and hydration and all other forms of health care to keep me alive.

1.4 WHEN AGENT'S AUTHORITY BECOMES EFFECTIVE.   Unless I otherwise specify in Exhibit "A", my agent's authority to make health care decisions for me takes effect immediately.

1.5 AGENT'S OBLIGATION.   My agent shall make health care decisions for me in accordance with this power of attorney for health care, any instructions I give in Part 2 of or Exhibit "A" to this form, and my other wishes to the extent known to my agent. To the extent my wishes are unknown, my agent shall make health care decisions for me in accordance with what my agent determines to be in my best interest. In determining my best interest, my agent shall consider my personal values to the extent known to my agent.

2.

1.6 AGENT'S POST -DEATH AUTHORITY. Unless I specify otherwise in Exhibit "A", my agent is authorized to make anatomical gifts, authorize an autopsy, and direct disposition of my remains.

PART 2: INSTRUCTIONS FOR HEALTH CARE

2.1 END-OF-LIFE DECISIONS. I direct that my health care providers and others involved in my care provide, withhold, or withdraw treatment in accordance with the choice I have marked below:

mwb **a. I Choose NOT To Prolong Life.** If I initial this line, I do **not** want my life to be prolonged and I do **not** want life-sustaining treatment to be provided or continued if **any** of the following conditions apply:

　　(1) I am in a coma or persistent vegetative state which two qualified physicians who are familiar with my condition, have diagnosed as irreversible (that is, there is no reasonable possibility that I will regain consciousness).

　　(2) I am terminally ill and the use of life sustaining procedures would only serve to artificially delay the moment of my death.

　　(3) I have an incurable and irreversible condition that will result in my death within a relatively short time.

　　(4) I become unconscious and, to a reasonable degree of medical certainty, I will not regain consciousness.

　　(5) The likely risks and burdens of treatment outweigh the expected benefits.
In such circumstances, I authorize my agent to sign a request to forego resuscitation measures, including a "do not resuscitate" ("DNR") form.

____ **b. I Choose To Prolong Life:** If I initial this line, I want my life to be prolonged as long as possible within the limits of generally accepted health care standards.

2.2 RELIEF FROM PAIN: Except as I state here, I direct that treatment for alleviation of pain or discomfort be provided at all times, even if it hastens my death:

mwb **a. NO RESTRICTIONS.** If l initial this line, no restrictions.

____ **b. RESTRICTIONS.** If l initial this line, the following restrictions: _____

_____
_____

(Add additional sheets if needed.)

3.

96

2.3 OTHER WISHES: I may attach special wishes and directions at Exhibit "A" attached to this instrument.

PART 3: DONATION OF ORGANS AT DEATH

____ **a. NO DONATIONS.** If I initial this line, I do NOT want any organs, tissues or parts donated following my death; **OR**

_Mᴜ__ **b. MAXIMUM DONATION AUTHORITY.** If I initial this line, I authorize my agent to give any needed organs, tissues, or parts following my death; **OR**

____ **c. LIMITED DONATION AUTHORITY.** If I initial this line, I give the following organs, tissues, or parts only following my death: _____
_____

____ **d. SPECIFIC PURPOSES.** If I initial this line and I have authorized any donations, my gift is for the following purposes only (1 will line through any of the following purposes that I do not want):

    (1) Transplant   (2) Therapy   (3) Research   (4) Education

PART 4: HIPAA RELEASE AUTHORITY

My agent has the authority to exercise the same rights as I would be able to exercise and shall be treated as I would be regarding the use and disclosure of my individually identifiable health information and medical records. This release authority applies to any information governed by the Health Insurance Portability and Accountability Act of 1996 (HIPAA), 42 USC 1320d and 45 CFR 160-164. I authorize any of the following entities that have provided treatment or services to me or that has paid for or is seeking payment from me for such services to give, disclose and release to my agent without restriction all of my individually identifiable health information and medical records:

    i. Physicians, dentists, medical or healthcare personnel;
    ii. Health plans, hospitals, clinics, laboratories, pharmacies, or other health care providers;
    iii. Any insurance company or other health care clearinghouses.

4.

The authority given my agent shall supersede any prior agreement that I have made with my health care providers to restrict access to or disclosure of my individually identifiable health information. The authority given my agent has no expiration date and shall expire only upon my explicit revocation in writing.

PART 5: EFFECT OF COPY
A copy of this form has the same effect as the original.

SIGNATURE

___9/3/09___   _Nora R. Harris_
(date)   (sign your name)

STATE OF CALIFORNIA   )
) ss.
COUNTY OF _SAN FRANCISCO_   )

On __September 3__, 2009, before me, _John J. Alkazin_____,

a Notary Public for California, personally appeared ____Nora R. Harris____, who

proved to me on the basis of satisfactory evidence to be the person whose name is subscribed

to the within instrument and acknowledged to me that she executed the same in her

authorized capacity, and that by her signature on the instrument the person or the entity upon

behalf of which the person acted, executed the instrument.

I certify under PENALTY OF PERJURY under the laws of State of California that

the foregoing paragraph is true and correct.

WITNESS my hand and official seal.

(seal)

_____
Notary Public for California

5.

Exhibit "A" to Advance Health Care Directive

I make the following special directions and statement of desires.

- **This Advance Directive becomes effective only upon my incapacity.** This instrument becomes effective only if
  -

*my primary physician signs a written statement that I am unable to make my own health care decisions.

*a board-certified psycho-neurologist or a board-certified psychiatrist, who is unrelated by blood or marriage to me, signs a written statement that he or she has examined me and that I lack the capacity to contract under the criteria set forth in California Probate Code Section 810 et. seq.

- **Restrictions on my agent's post-death authority.**
  -

*My agent may authorize an autopsy (California Health & Safety Code Section 7113).
*My agent may direct disposition of my remains.
*My agent is authorized and directed to handle the disposition of my remains in accordance with the directions contained in my Last Will and Testament or as otherwise communicated to my agent.

- **Medical Care.** In addition to general authorities, my agent is specifically authorized to:
*Request, review and receive any information, verbal or written, regarding my physical or mental health, including (but not limited to) medical and hospital records; sign on my behalf any releases or other documents that may be required to obtain this information; and consent to disclosure of this information.
*Sign on my behalf documents purporting to be "Refusal to Permit Treatment", "Leaving Hospital Against Medical Advice", "Do Not Resuscitate (DNR)" and "No Code" or similar instructions, and to sign any waiver or release from liability reasonably required by a hospital or physician.
*Consent to X-ray examinations and anesthesia.

- **Extent of Agent's Authority.** My agent shall have the broadest discretion possible during any period that I am incapable of giving informed consent about my medical care, which shall include consenting to, withdrawing consent to, any treatment, service, or procedure to diagnose, maintain or treat any physical or mental condition of mine. Unless I line through any power listed below, this authority shall include:
*Artificial respiration (commencement or termination) .
*Artificial nutrition and hydration (nourishment provided by feeding tube) (commencement or termination).
*Cardiopulmonary resuscitation (CPR).
*Antibiotics.
*Organ transplantations.

6.

99

*Blood transfusions.
*Other treatments.

- **What my agent may NOT do.** I acknowledge that California law provides that my agent may **not** do any of the following without a court order:
-
*Commitment or placement in a mental health treatment facility against my objection.
*Consent to convulsive treatment as defined in Welfare and Institutions Code Section 5325.
*Consent to psychosurgery as defined in Welfare and Institutions Code Section 5324).
*Consent to sterilization.
*Consent to abortion.

- **Determining where I may live.**
-
* I wish to live in my home for as long as reasonably possible without endangering my physical or mental health and safety, or my financial security. My agent is authorized to hire whatever household employees or personal care givers as may be necessary to permit me to live in my home.
* If my agent determines that it is inappropriate or dangerous for me to live in my home, then I desire the least restrictive and most home-like environment deemed appropriate by my agent, to include (but not be limited to) residential facilities, hospitals, hospices, nursing homes, convalescent facilities, and private board and care facilities. I wish to live as close as possible to my residence, so that I may still visit friends and neighbors to the extent that my agent determines that I will benefit from those relationships. I ask that my agent allow me as much autonomy and privacy as possible, including placement in an assisted living care facility or board and care facility. I desire that my agent encourage me in my social relationships and social interaction even if I seem no longer able to recognize my family and friends or to fully participate in social activities.
* I wish to return home as soon as possible after any hospitalization or convalescent care.

- **Visitation rights.** My agent shall have the first right of visitation while I am a patient in a hospital, health care facility, or other institution, including (but not limited to) any intensive care or coronary care unit of a medical facility. My agent shall have the right to restrict other visitors if my agent determines that is necessary for my health.

- **Employment and discharge of others.** My agent shall have the power to employ and discharge physicians, dentists, nurses, therapists, household employees and other persons as my agent determines necessary or proper for my physical, mental and emotional well being. My agent shall arrange for my transportation and meals; shall handle my mail; and shall arrange for my recreation and entertainment. My agent shall have the right to arrange for reasonable compensation for these persons, and to charge these expenses to my trust or other assets.

- **Psychiatric care.** If two independent psychiatrists licensed to practice in the State of California examine me and determine that I am in immediate need of hospitalization or institutionalization because of mental disorders, alcoholism or substance abuse, then my

7.

agent shall have the authority to arrange for my voluntary admission to an appropriate hospital or institution for treatment of the diagnosed problem or disorder; to arrange for and consent to private psychiatric and psychological treatment for me; and to refuse consent for any such hospitalization or treatment; and to revoke consent for any such hospitalization or treatment that my agent or I may have given at a prior time.

- **Life prolonging procedures**. My agent is authorized to request that aggressive medical therapy be instituted or discontinued, including (but not limited to) cardiopulmonary resuscitation, cardiac pacemaker, renal dialysis, parental feeding, the use of respirators and ventilators, blood transfusions, nasogastric tube use, intravenous feeding, and endotracheal tube use.

8.

Please note the red arrows which identify the pertinent parts of the advance directive that guided my instructions. The last paragraph (above) created the legal dispute over "spoon-feeding." Notice the specific language:

My agent is authorized to request aggressive medical therapy be instituted or **discontinued**, …renal dialysis, **parental feeding**, the use of respirators and ventilators, blood transfusions, nasogastric tube use, *intravenous feeding*, and endotracheal tube use.

We took *parental feeding* to be spoon-feeding. The court indicated that "parental feeding" was really parenteral feeding which is:

Parenteral feeding is the intravenous administration of nutrients. This may be supplemental to oral or **tube feeding**, or it may provide the only source of **nutrition** as total **parenteral nutrition** (TPN). Oct. 21, 2014.[84]

The State of California removed this from the advance directive in its next edition.

The reason I included the document was to show that major ethical issues are derived from the advance directive: how the maker of the directive wants to be treated when they cannot feed themselves, regardless of reason; the use of life-prolonging medicines when the disease enters its later stages; remaining in the home rather than placement; and if placement, in "... the least restrictive and home-like environment"; and the use of pain medications, which may shorten life.

Additional Ethical Issues

The above is not an exhaustive list. There are additional issues not part of the advance directive, such as dying at home rather than a facility. The ethical issue here: what is *your* desire? You have been in mourning for years—the care receiver does not recognize you or mistakes you for someone else. They are not able to communicate or even understand where they are or the environment they are in. So, the question is, do you bring them home or let them pass in the facility?

My recommendation is to do whatever reduces your stress. If it's letting them pass in a facility, then do it. If you *must* follow their wishes then be as simple as possible. Remember, what you do at home is for *you*, not the care receiver, as they will not understand their surroundings nor be able to verbally communicate with family or friends. You will have to work with hospice as the end approaches; the nurse will be administering morphine and sedatives to calm the care receiver. You will have to notify the mortuary to remove the body.

84

https://www.google.com/search?source=hp&ei=EzvXXerMEdeS0PEPv82OiAk&q=parental+feeding&oq=parental+feeding&gs_l=psy-ab.3..0i10j0l2j0i10l3j0j0i10l3.2151.6699..12052...0.0..0.169.1836.2j14......0....1..gws-wiz.......0i13

1.L8eTCemsj7c&ved=0ahUKEwiqoqzJ1vzlAhVXCTQIHb-mA5EQ4dUDCAc&uact=5

My Experience

I let Nora pass in the facility. The facility caregivers worked with hospice and the mortuary. They also washed the body before the mortician came. I found this to be better for me. I watched the whole process without having to call or communicate with the mortuary or wash the body, which I did not know how to do.

Nora's passing was a great relief for me and her. I felt the less involvement from me was better. My therapist helped me to deal with the feelings of guilt and remorse. He made me realize that it was not necessary for me to do all this at home. The staff at the memory care facility had more experience and were better able to manage the immediate aftermath of Nora's passing.

When Nora was diagnosed, she volunteered to provide her brain and spine to UCSF for research. UCSF and the mortuary worked out the details in advance and it was accomplished without involving me, definitely a relief. Her remains were cremated by the mortuary, as per her wishes.

CHAPTER 9: PLACING A LOVED ONE

As the disease progresses, you become more a guardian than a spouse or child of the care receiver. As they become more incapable of making rational decisions, managing the finances, taking care of themselves, you become a guardian.

You may be thinking about placing, or have already placed, the care receiver in a facility. If you have run out of patience in caregiving, it does not matter where or what stage the care receiver is in—it is time to place them into an environment that is designed for their care, such as a memory care facility.

Becoming a Guardian

There comes a point when you need to be a guardian, not a caregiver. The caregiving should be done by others. You have done your job well, and the rational thing to do is to place the care receiver in a facility structured to take care of patients with dementia and Alzheimer's disease. A legal guardianship may be a requirement of the facility where you are placing them. This is to protect the care receiver, memory care facility, and even you from a feud over whether it is proper to place the person in such a facility.

Legal Reporting

If you are awarded guardianship, there are reporting requirements to state agencies dictated by state regulations. I found it was a great benefit to go to the bank and set up an account for the sole purpose of paying guardianship expenses. I also found that this was a great mechanism for keeping financial records of the guardianship. The beginning and ending balances of the guardianship account on bank statements made it easy to summarize the expenses for the year. I paid for the memory care facility, doctors, supplies, clothes, and other incidental expenses out of this account. I periodically funded the account from other sources (income, retirement accounts, stock sales). And if there ever were to be a legal dispute over the efficacy of the guardianship, bank statements are a great legal mechanism for proving financial adherence to law and the prudent person rule.

Placement & Guilt

In support groups, the most guilt-ridden process was placing a loved one in a facility. Most people are very reluctant to place the person. That is why we continually repeated the mantra: It is not where the care receiver is, it is where you, the caregiver, are! If you have run out of patience in caregiving, it does not matter what stage the care receiver is in; it is time to place them into an environment designed for their care, such as a memory care facility. This is taking care of yourself as it is giving you the relief you need to survive. If you are succumbing to the stress, you need to change the situation.

However, *guilt* is the major factor in not placing a loved one in a memory care facility. The guilt here is two-fold: one is guilt over wedding vows, "till death do us part ..." and "in sickness and in health ..." ring especially loud in the ears of caregivers, or a partner or child promised they would take care of them. These commitments are interpreted by some caregivers as:

- I *must* take care of them at home, by myself
- I am not meeting my vows and commitments if I place them
- It means that I do not love them enough or I am rejecting them
- They will be very mad at me
- It makes me feel heartless or cruel because I am locking them up

Second, guilt over placing them in a secure facility is like sending them to prison. It is depressing when you take a tour and think, "I would not want to be put here."

This is where a therapist can be a great help. A caregiver should understand that it is not where the care receiver is, it is where the caregiver is. If the caregiver can't take it anymore, it is time to place, regardless the care receiver's perceived capabilities to stay at home. Remember, the stress of caregiving contributes to the death of four out of 10 caregivers before the person they are caregiving passes.

My Experience

My therapist really helped me to place Nora and to understand why. I was working from home and she would constantly come up to me and start conversations, even when I was on a conference call. She had progressed to where the person I married was gone. He also made me understand my guilt was coming from actions taken or not taken when I was growing up.

Placing a Loved One

Placement is one of the hardest decisions to make or implement, because it fundamentally changes the caregiver situation. The care receiver is no longer in the house. Generally, they are not coming home, they will pass in the facility.

The caregiver should have made nonnegotiable criteria for placement in the early part of this journey. What do I mean by that? Simply put, criteria that can be objectively observed and easily identified. And the caregiver cannot argue with themselves when the behavior occurs.

This concept of unnegotiability came from when I was managing programmers at the bank. When we had a software problem that was affecting the public, we wanted to fix it as soon as possible. I would ask the engineer who wrote the code how long they thought it would take to find the problem and fix it. They would say *Give me a half hour* to identify the specific code causing the problem. I said okay. In a half hour, I would go back and ask if they found the code problem. They would say *Give me another half hour*. I would agree and return in a half hour. If they said *I need another half hour* I would say, *Okay, but if you have not found the problem when I come back, I will ask others to come help work on the problem*. There is a natural tendency to say *I can handle* this and *just give me a little more time*.

This is also true with caregiving. *I can handle this, I promised. I am doing fine; I need just a little help. I view placing as a failure on my part as a caregiver.* Interestingly, it is a failure on the part of the caregiver if they do *not* get substantial help in caregiving, such as placement or live-in help. The nonnegotiable criteria should be developed by the caregiver and, if possible, the care receiver at time of diagnosis and in its aftermath discussion. Involving the care receiver is touchy, as they may not be really capable of participating in such a discussion. This can also be part of the advance directive conversation. You may find that the care receiver is very concerned about your future and/or finances.

Some behaviors that one is not capable of tolerating or care for are:

- Violence
- Incontinence
- Excessive dependence
- Lack of sleep
- Hostility
- "Can't take it anymore"
- Interference

My nonnegotiable criteria was incontinence and, later, interference and interruptions with my job. If I did not work, I couldn't pay for her care—a nonnegotiable.

Placement Options

At-home care may be the only option because of the lack of local resources or the inability to pay for a facility. All care is the responsibility of the caregiver, even for obtaining outside help, much like a hiring process. You interview caregivers and select one that seems to fit your criteria. You are also responsible for managing their help. You determine the scope, hours, expectations, and activities that the outside help is responsible for. Ideally, it should be 24/7. This option deals with guilt better than the others.

If you do have 24/7 help, do the cost benefit analysis on this option versus placement, as it will probably turn out to be more expensive than the cost of a facility. And do not forget to include your time and effort in the cost/benefit assessment. Another factor: many professional caregivers are not trained to deal with dementia or Alzheimer's disease. This puts an added burden on you.

Assisted living, in my opinion, is not really an option for placement, maybe just an option for early stages of the disease. It is really *independent living* in a managed environment. There may be nursing assistance available, but the mission of assisted living is making the person as independent as possible. This is not suited to persons with dementia or Alzheimer's disease. However, many the assisted living facilities are paired with a memory care facility, which means the person in assisted living will be moved into the memory care facility at some point. Major care decisions are the responsibility of the caregiver who is highly involved in the care of the loved one. This can be both a plus and a minus.

A foster home is where a multibedroom house, generally four to six rooms, is turned into a care facility. It is simulating care in your home with a small, dedicated staff. The description of a foster home by the State of Oregon is as follows.

When elderly people or adults with physical disabilities are no longer able to care for themselves in their own homes, adult foster care may be an option. Adult foster homes are single-family residences that offer 24-hour care in a home-like setting. A wide variety of residents are served in adult foster homes, from those needing only room,

122

board, and minimal personal assistance to those residents needing full personal care, or skilled nursing care with the help of community-based registered nurses.[85]

Adult foster care in Oregon limits residences to five occupants. Homes that care for a greater number are called residential care facilities (RCF). Medicaid: the Aged & Physically Disabled Waiver covers personal care and support services in both types of locations. The newer K Plan does as well.[86]

From the state of Virginia, the definition of a foster home is:

"Adult foster care" means room and board, supervision, and special services to an adult who has a physical or mental condition. Adult foster care may be provided by a single provider for up to three adults.[87]

Adult foster care is defined as care homes for three or fewer residents. While no Medicaid program was found to serve that type of residence, larger residences can receive Medicaid reimbursement through the soon to expire, Alzheimer's Assisted Living Waiver. As of writing it was uncertain whether the new Commonwealth Coordinated Care (CCC) Plus Medicaid Waiver will offer this benefit.[88]

[NOTE] If there are more than three adults, the foster home will need to be licensed by the state of Virginia.

The owner or manager of the foster home must live in the home where they are generally providing care for elderly people, either rehabilitation or for their remaining life. Many people like this approach because it feels like a home. However, there are major issues for people with dementia or Alzheimer's disease with foster homes. The primary one is they are not designed or equipped to handle dementia or Alzheimer's patients. They may lack security or doors that cannot be opened by the residents. The staff may be inexperienced in taking care of Alzheimer's patients.

In a support group, there was a person who placed his wife in a foster home. She spent her day trying to get out and was continually leaving the house and trying to open the gates around the property. The facility had to place special locks on doors and gates to

---

85 https://www.oregon.gov/dhs/providers-partners/licensing/APD-AFH/Pages/Overview.aspx
86 https://www.payingforseniorcare.com/medicaid-waivers/adult-foster-care
87 https://law.justia.com/codes/virginia/2017/title-63.2/chapter-1/section-63.2-100/
88 https://www.payingforseniorcare.com/medicaid-waivers/adult-foster-care

keep her inside. This prevented the other non-dementia residents from going outside and sitting on the patio or deck and the cost of the locks was charged to her husband. Soon afterward she was moved to a memory care facility.

The State of Oregon defines a **memory care facility**:

Memory care communities provide specialized services in a secured environment for individuals with dementia. These rules are designed to ensure that residents living in memory care communities have positive quality of life, consumer protection, and person directed care. Resident's rights, dignity, choice, comfort, and independence are promoted in this setting.[89]

The State of Virginia defines a memory care facility:

In Virginia regulations, memory care is called **"special care units" within assisted living residences**. These communities are specifically for people with Alzheimer's disease or related dementia, providing personal and healthcare services, 24-hour supervision, social and recreational activities, and anything else in residents' personal service plans. Staff needs to be trained to provide assistance with activities of daily living, like eating and bathing, and instrumental activities of daily living, like managing money or medications.[90] [Emphasis added]

These facilities are specifically designed to care for people with dementia or Alzheimer's disease. They must be lockdown facilities where the residents cannot leave the appropriate areas and have staff who are specifically trained to care for residents with dementia or Alzheimer's disease.

The main issue with these facilities is the expense; which keeps deserving people out. Many of these facilities, though, will help in getting Medicaid to pay for the care. If the state supports it, Medicaid has specific language that allows for payment to memory care facilities (and other places like nursing homes) in the Affordable Care Act (ACA). If the ACA is repealed or revoked, this goes away.

The state regulates all of these options: assisted living, foster homes, and memory care facilities, monitoring them through a team of paid and volunteer ombudsmen who regularly visit each facility and ensure it is meeting all state requirements, rules, and

---

89 http://www.dhs.state.or.us/policy/spd/rules/411_057.pdf
90 https://www.dementiacarecentral.com/memory-care/virginia

regulations. They are also on the lookout for elder abuse and can report an institution to the state which can then restrict new patient admissions or shut the facility down.

At-home care may not be regulated or audited by the state, but if a complaint about a home care situation is filed with the ombudsmen agency, the state can come in an evaluate the complaint as an elder abuse issue.

My Experience

I placed Nora in a memory care facility that was specifically designed for Alzheimer's patients. It was designed as a hub and spoke arrangement; four spokes off of the hub— the residences were at the end of each spoke. Every spoke had a common dining area, kitchenette, and nurses' station along with about 10 bedrooms, most double occupancy. The complex had a main kitchen which provided the meals to the residences. A central meeting area and administrative offices were outside of the locked hub and residences. All of the staff were trained in dementia care and there was a registered nurse on duty 24/7. A doctor visited the complex once a week to review and see patients.

When I placed Nora, she soon took up walking around the hub and going into the residences, coming and going around the hub again. Constantly. This behavior was not exhibited at home. I rejected foster homes and assisted living because of the wandering issue of and her "I do not want to be here" attitude. She was in the memory care facility from January 2013 to October 2017.

Selecting the Facility

Your nonnegotiable criteria have been met and it is time to find a facility for your loved one. I created a spreadsheet of the requirements which I thought were necessary for placement. There were two parts: one part was my requirements, and the other part was what I thought were requirements for Nora. The major categories were: family involvement, staffing, program and services, residents, environment, meals, policies and procedures, cost, and intangibles. See the sample spreadsheet below with the requirements in the left column; the other columns can be filled out as you visit and compare facilities.

Topic	Your Requirements	Placement 1	Placement 2	Placement3
Family Involvement				
Families are encouraged to participate in care planning				
Families are informed of changes in resident's condition and care needs				
Families are encouraged to communicate with staff				
Staffing				
Medical Care is provided				
Facility manages medicines, including ordering				
Is there a doctor that has weekly (monthly?) visits?				
Accept Private Health insurance for Medical Costs (or Medicare/Medicaid)				
Personal Care and assistance is provided				
Staff recognize persons with dementia as unique individuals, and care is personalized to meet specific needs, abilities and interests				
Staff is trained in dementia care				
Number of staff on duty during graveyard shift				

Topic	Your Requirements	Placement 1	Placement 2	Placement 3
Program and Services				
Appropriate services and programming based on specific health and behavioral care needs are available				
Planned activities that take place (ask to see activity schedule; note if the activity listed at the time of your visit is occurring)				
Activities are available on the weekends or during evenings				
Activities are designed to meet specific needs, interests and abilities				
Transportation is available for medical appointments and shopping for personal items				
Care planning sessions are held regularly				
Residents				
Personal care is done with respect and dignity				
Residents are comfortable, relaxed, and involved in activities				
Residents are well groomed, clean, and dressed appropriately				
Environment				
Indoor space allows for freedom of movement and promotes independence				
Indoor and outdoor areas are safe and secure				
The facility is easy to navigate				
There is a designated family visiting area				
Resident rooms are clean and spacious				
Residents are allowed to bring familiar items with them, such as photos, bedding, a chair, etc.				

Topic	Your Requirements	Placement 1	Placement 2	Placement 3
Meals				
There are regular meal and snack times				
Food is appetizing (ask to see the weekly menu and come for a meal)				
The dining environment is pleasant				
Family and friends are able to join at mealtime				
Staff have a plan for monitoring adequate nutrition				
Staff are able to provide for any special dietary needs				
Staff provide appropriate assistance based on person's abilities (for example, encouragement during meals or assisted feeding in advanced stages)				
There are no environmental distractions during meal time (noisy TV, etc.)				
Policies and Procedures				
Do they require guardianship?				
Is the facility only for dementia residents or is there a mixture				
Family and friends are able to participate in care				
Visiting hours work for the family				
Discharge policy has been discussed (learn about any situation or condition that would lead to a discharge from the facility, such as change in behavior or financial circumstances)				

Topic	Your Requirements	Placement 1	Placement 2	Placement 3
Cost				
Monthly fee				
Additional Costs				
medicines				
doctor visits				
supplies				
Special treatment (shower/bath assistance, etc.)				
Accept Medicare/Medicaid				
Accept Private Insurance (Long Term Care)				
Accept Private Health insurance for Medical Costs				
Ownership (one person, consortium, corporation) and financial soundness				
Accept Credit Cards/electronic payments				
Intangibles				
During the tour, is there friendly/loving physical contact by staff towards residents, such as pat on back, touch on the shoulder, resident hugs the tour guide, etc.)				
Does the person that is showing you around know the residents by name, talk to them?				
How long have they been in this location and in business?				
Fire drills? / Safety drills?				

I used this in my selection process. On one tour, I noticed the person leading it never spoke to, touched, or interacted with the residents. On a tour of a different facility, the person leading the tour knew each resident's name and would give them hugs; residents would come up to her and interact. Two completely different cultural experiences. It is part of the intangibles section in the spreadsheet. Obviously, I choose the second place over the first.

One needs to also look at cost closely, not so much as to how much, but as to how it is structured. One place had a lower base rate, but three to four tiers of care, and each caried an incremental cost added to the base rate. For example, the base level of care might be $3,500. The first level of care might be the minimum care: meals, medicines, laundry, etc., for $1,000. The second level might add special care items, like changing bandages, giving shots, or special diets, etc. This level of care would be $1,500 on top of the $3,500 per month. And so on. Other facilities may have a flat, inclusive fee. For example, I paid $4,800 for double occupancy, which included all care—whether it was minimal or involved feeding, bathing, etc.

From a budgeting standpoint, I preferred the flat fee approach because it would not increase over time as the care became more complex. I also liked the idea of a doctor coming to the facility once a week. I did not want to be responsible for taking Nora to the doctor for routine medical care. I also found that an unintended consequence of a doctor coming to the facility was the recommendation of hospice care. The first time was because of Nora's loss of weight over the six- to eight-week period. I would not have taken Nora to the doctor every week, so the weight loss would not have been seen as a medical issue.

These are just a few items you want to evaluate as you compare places. One more thing: I do not think it is a good idea to discuss placement with the person, bring them along for the visit, discuss the comparisons, or the timing of the placement. It does not serve any purpose for you, nor does it provide comfort to the loved one/care receiver. If anything, it will make them more anxious.

How do you place them if they do not want to go? Nora didn't. The answer is *you lie*. We learn to tell untruths a lot when coping with this disease. "No, I do not know where the car keys are." "No, I do not know why the power tools do not work." And so on. Placing is another one of these occasions. Nora repeatedly said she did not want to go into a memory care center.

When the time came, I told her that I had to go on a business trip and could not find someone who would stay with her for three days. However, I found a place she could go while I was on the business trip and when I returned, I would get her and we would go home.

She did not like it, but went along with it. I took her to the memory care place and they came out to meet us and took Nora by the hand and led her into the facility and to her residence. I said I would be back soon. I then left (without seeing her to her room) and drove to the Bay Area for a week. Not to work, but to see friends. Going away was at the suggestion of the memory care facility staff.

After you place your loved one, then what? You have to reintegrate yourself into society.

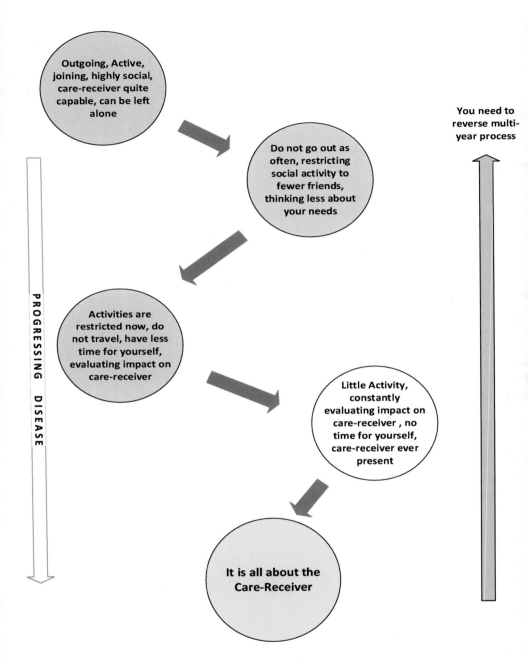

FIGURE 8: IMPACT ON RELATIONSHIPS

When you first place your loved one, you need to go out of town for a week or two, visit friends or relatives, for two reasons:

- It lets the diagnosed adjust to their new surroundings
- It lets you adjust to your new situation and understand how involved you were in caregiving

You are not abandoning them. You are providing the best care for them—care that you determined you could no longer provide. That is why you placed them.

Second, do not visit or have meals with them every day, for two reasons:

- It lets the diagnosed adjust to their new surroundings and routine
- It lets you adjust to your new situation and understand how involved you were in caregiving

Let them get familiar with their daily routine (including meals) and with the other residents. Your presence is a reminder that they are inside and you are outside. You will be seen as a way out. In addition, you need to understand how far you were from a normal social life.

Third, **they are leaving you**, you are not leaving them. The disease is taking them away from you. Their memory of you is fading and will vanish. They will not differentiate you from some other person or family member. This is not your fault. You did not cause this.

You have a life to live—you need to put yourself first now, not them. They are being well cared for, you are not. You did your job. You need to reintegrate yourself into society. You need to have physical contact with others, such as a dinner with someone, without your spouse or partner. There is a lot of life yet to live.

Three people in my support group have married since the passing of their spouse or partner.

There is a lot of life left to live!

ADVANCE DIRECTIVES

Oregon Advance Directive

Idaho Advance Directive

Washington Advance Directive

Washington Dementia Advance Directive

Virginia Advance Directive

ADVANCE DIRECTIVE (STATE OF OREGON)

This form may be used in Oregon to choose a person to make health care decisions for you if you cannot speak for yourself. The person is called a health care representative. If you do not have an effective health care representative appointed and cannot speak for yourself, a health care representative will be appointed for you in the order of priority set forth in ORS 127.635(2).

This form also allows you to express your values and beliefs with respect to health care decisions and your preferences for health care.

1. If you have completed an advance directive in the past, this new advance directive will replace any older directive.

2. You must sign this form for it to be effective. You must also have it witnessed by two witnesses or a notary. Your appointment of a health care representative is not effective until the health care representative accepts the appointment.

3. If your advance directive includes directions regarding the withdrawal of life support or tube feeding, you may revoke your advance directive at any time and in any manner that expresses your desire to revoke it.

4. In all other cases, you may revoke your advance directive at any time and in any manner as long as you are capable of making medical decisions.

1. ABOUT ME.

Name: _____ Date of Birth: _____

Telephone numbers: (Home)_____(Work)_____(Cell)_____

Address: _____

Email: _____

2. MY HEALTH CARE REPRESENTATIVE.

I choose the following person as my health care representative to make health care decisions for me if I can't speak for myself.

Name:_____ Relationship: _____

Telephone numbers: (Home)_____(Work)_____(Cell)_____

Address: _____

Email: _____

I choose the following people to be my alternate health care representatives if my first choice is not available to make health care decisions for me or if I cancel the first health care representative's appointment.

First alternate health care representative:

Name: _____ Relationship: _____
Telephone numbers: (Home)_____(Work)_____(Cell)_____
Address: _____
   Email: _____

Second alternate health care representative:

Name: _____ Relationship: _____
Telephone numbers: (Home)_____(Work)_____(Cell)_____
Address: _____
   Email: _____

3. INSTRUCTIONS TO MY HEALTH CARE REPRESENTATIVE.
If you wish to give instructions to your health care representative about your health care decisions, initial one of the following three statements:

_____ To the extent appropriate, my health care representative must follow my instructions.

_____ My instructions are guidelines for my health care representative to consider when making decisions about my care.

_____ Other instructions: _____

4. DIRECTIONS REGARDING MY END-OF-LIFE CARE.
In filling out these directions, keep the following in mind:

- The term "as my health care provider recommends" means that you want your health care provider to use life support if they believe it could be helpful and that you want them to discontinue life support if they believe it is not helping your health condition or symptoms.
  The term "life support" means any medical treatment that maintains life by sustaining, restoring or replacing a vital function.

135

- The term "tube feeding" means artificially administered food and water.
- If you refuse tube feeding, you should understand that malnutrition, dehydration, and death will probably result.
- You will receive care for your comfort and cleanliness no matter what choices you make.

A. **Statement Regarding End-of-Life Care**. You may initial the statement below if you agree with it. If you initial the statement you may, but do not have to, list one or more conditions for which you do not want to receive life support.

_____ I do not want my life to be prolonged by life support. I also do not want tube feeding as life support. I want my health care provider to allow me to die naturally if they and another knowledgeable health care provider confirm I am in any of the medical conditions listed below.

B. **Additional Directions Regarding End-of-Life Care**. Here are my desires about my health care if my health care provider and another knowledgeable health care provider confirm that I am in a medical condition described below:

a. Close to Death. If I am close to death and life support would only postpone my death,

INITIAL ONE:
_____ I want to receive tube feeding.
_____ I want tube feeding only as my health care provider recommends.
_____ I DO NOT WANT tube feeding.

INITIAL ONE:
_____ I want any other life support that may apply.
_____ I want life support only as my health care provider recommends.
_____ I DO NOT WANT life support.

b. Permanently Unconscious. If I am unconscious and it is very unlikely that I will ever become conscious again:

INITIAL ONE:
_____ I want to receive tube feeding.
_____ I want tube feeding only as my health care provider recommends.
_____ I DO NOT WANT tube feeding.

INITIAL ONE:
_____ I want any other life support that may apply.
_____ I want life support only as my health care provider recommends.
_____ I DO NOT WANT life support.

c. Advanced Progressive Illness. If I have a progressive, fatal illness in an advanced stage and I am consistently and permanently unable to communicate by any means, swallow food and water safely, care for myself and recognize my family and other people, and it is very unlikely that my condition will substantially improve:

INITIAL ONE:

_____ I want to receive tube feeding.
_____ I want tube feeding only as my health care provider recommends.
_____ I DO NOT WANT tube feeding.

INITIAL ONE:

_____ I want any other life support that may apply.
_____ I want life support only as my health care provider recommends.
_____ I DO NOT WANT life support.

d. Extraordinary Suffering. If life support would not help my medical condition and would make me suffer permanent and severe pain:
INITIAL ONE:

_____ I want to receive tube feeding.
_____ I want tube feeding only as my health care provider recommends.
_____ I DO NOT WANT tube feeding.

INITIAL ONE:

_____ I want any other life support that may apply.
_____ I want life support only as my health care provider recommends.
_____ I DO NOT WANT life support.

C. **Additional Instructions.** You may attach to this document any writing or recording of your values and beliefs related to health care decisions. These attachments will serve as guidelines for health care providers. Attachments may include a description of what you would like to happen if you are close to death, if you are permanently unconscious, if you have an advanced progressive illness or if you are suffering permanent and severe pain.

5. MY SIGNATURE.

My signature: _____   Date: _____

6. WITNESS.
COMPLETE EITHER A OR B WHEN YOU SIGN.

A. NOTARY:

State of _____

County of _____

Signed or attested before me on_____, 2_____, by_____.

_____
Notary Public - State of Oregon

B. WITNESS DECLARATION:

The person completing this form is personally known to me or has provided proof of identity, has signed or acknowledged the person's signature on the document in my presence and appears to be not under duress and to understand the purpose and effect of this form. In addition, I am not the person's health care representative or alternative health care representative, and I am not the person's attending health care provider.

Witness Name (print): _____

Signature: _____   Date:_____

Witness Name (print): _____

Signature: _____Date: _____

7. ACCEPTANCE BY MY HEALTH CARE REPRESENTATIVE.
I accept this appointment and agree to serve as health care representative.

Health care representative: _____

Printed name: _____

Signature or other verification of acceptance: _____
Date: _____

First alternate health care representative:

Printed name: _____

Signature or other verification of acceptance: _____
Date: _____

Second alternate health care representative:

Printed name: _____

Signature or other verification of acceptance: _____
Date: _____

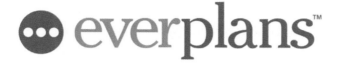

NOTE: This form is being provided to you as a public service. The attached forms are provided "as is" and are not the substitute for the advice of an attorney. By providing these forms and information, Everplans is not providing legal advice to you. Consult an attorney if you need legal advice of any nature.

Read more and get more forms at Everplans' Advance Directive page.

LIVING WILL AND DURABLE POWER OF ATTORNEY FOR HEALTH CARE

Date of Directive: _____

Name of person executing Directive: _____

Address of person executing Directive: _____

_____

A Living Will

A Directive to Withhold or to Provide Treatment

1.   I willfully and voluntarily make known my desire that my life shall not be prolonged artificially under the circumstances set forth below. This Directive shall be effective only if I am unable to communicate my instructions and:

    a.   I have an incurable or irreversible injury, disease, illness or condition, and a medical doctor who has examined me has certified:

        1.   That such injury, disease, illness or condition is terminal; and

        2.   That the application of artificial life-sustaining procedures would serve only to prolong my life artificially; and

        3.   That my death is imminent, whether or not artificial life-sustaining procedures are utilized.

OR

    b.   I have been diagnosed as being in a persistent vegetative state.

In such event, I direct that the following marked expression of my intent be followed and that I receive any medical treatment or care that may be required to keep me free of pain or distress.

Check one box and initial the line after such box:

☐ _____ I direct that all medical treatment, care, and procedures necessary to to restore my health and sustain my life be provided to me. Nutrition and hydration, whether artificial or non-artificial, shall not be withheld or withdrawn from me if I would likely die primarily from malnutrition or dehydration rather than from my injury, disease, illness or condition.

141

☐ _____ I direct that all medical treatment, care and procedures, including artificial life-sustaining procedures, be withheld or withdrawn, except that nutrition and hydration, whether artificial or non-artificial shall not be withheld or withdrawn from me if, as a result, I would likely die primarily from malnutrition or dehydration rather than from my injury, disease, illness or condition, as follows:
(If none of the following boxes are checked and initialed, then both nutrition and hydration, of any nature, whether artificial or non-artificial, shall be administered.)

Check <u>one</u> box and initial the line after such box:

☐ _____ A.   Only hydration of any nature, whether artificial or non- artificial, shall be administered.

☐ _____ B.   Only nutrition, of any nature, whether artificial or non- artificial, shall be administered.

☐ _____ C.   Both nutrition and hydration, of any nature, whether artificial or non-artificial shall be administered.

OR

☐ _____ I direct that all medical treatment, care and procedures be withheld or withdrawn, including withdrawal of the administration of artificial nutrition and hydration.

2.   If I have been diagnosed as pregnant, this Directive shall have no force during the course of my pregnancy.

3.   I understand the full importance of this Directive and am mentally competent to make this Directive. No participant in the making of this Directive or in its being carried into effect shall be held responsible in any way for complying with my directions.

4.   Check <u>one</u> box and initial the line after such box:

☐ _____ I have discussed these decisions with my physician and have also completed a Physician Orders for Scope of Treatment (POST) form that contains directions that may be more specific than, but are compatible with, this Directive. I hereby approve of those orders and incorporate them herein as if fully set forth.

OR

☐ _____ I have not completed a Physician Orders for Scope of Treatment (POST) form. If a POST form is later signed by my physician, then this living will shall be deemed modified to be compatible with the terms of the POST form.

A Durable Power of Attorney for Health Care

DESIGNATION OF HEALTH CARE AGENT

None of the following may be designated as your agent:

(1) your treating health care provider;

(2) a non-relative employee of your treating health care provider;

(3) an operator of a community care facility; or

(4) a non-relative employee of an operator of a community care facility.

If the agent or an alternate agent designated in this Directive is my spouse, and our marriage is thereafter dissolved, such designation shall be thereupon revoked.

I do hereby designate and appoint the following individual as my attorney in fact (agent) to make health care decisions for me as authorized in this Directive.

(Insert name, address and telephone number of one individual only as your agent to make health care decisions for you.)

Name of Health Care Agent: _____

Address of Health Care Agent: _____

Telephone Number of Health Care Agent: _____

For the purposes of this Directive, "health care decision" means consent, refusal of consent, or withdrawal of consent to any care, treatment, service, or procedure to maintain, diagnose or treat an individual's physical condition.

143

CREATION OF DURABLE POWER OF ATTORNEY FOR HEALTH CARE

By this portion of this Directive, I create a durable power of attorney for health care. This power of attorney shall not be affected by my subsequent incapacity. This power shall be effective only when I am unable to communicate rationally.

1. GENERAL STATEMENT OF AUTHORITY GRANTED

I hereby grant to my agent full power and authority to make health care decisions for me to the same extent that I could make such decisions for myself if I had the capacity to do so. In exercising this authority, my agent shall make health care decisions that are consistent with my desires as stated in this Directive or otherwise made known to my agent including, but not limited to, my desires concerning obtaining or refusing or withdrawing artificial life-sustaining care, treatment, services and procedures, including such desires set forth in a living will, Physician Orders for Scope of Treatment (POST) form, or similar document executed by me, if any.

(If you want to limit the authority of your agent to make health care decisions for you, you can state the limitations in paragraph 4, "Statement of Desires, Special Provisions, and Limitations," below. You can indicate your desires by including a statement of your desires in the same paragraph.)

2. STATEMENT OF DESIRES, SPECIAL PROVISIONS, AND LIMITATIONS

(Your agent must make health care decisions that are consistent with your known desires. You can, but are not required to, state your desires in the space provided below. You should consider whether you want to include a statement of your desires concerning artificial life-sustaining care, treatment, services and procedures. You can also include a statement of your desires concerning other matters relating to your health care, including a list of one or more persons whom you designate to be able to receive medical information about you and/or to be allowed to visit you in a medical institution. You can also make your desires known to your agent by discussing your desires with your agent or by some other means. If there are any types of treatment that you do not want to be used, you should state them in the space below. If you want to limit in any other way the authority given your agent by this Directive, you should state the limits in the space below. If you do not state any limits, your agent will have broad powers to make health care decisions for you, except to the extent that there are limits provided by law.)

In exercising the authority under this durable power of attorney for health care, my agent shall act consistently with my desires as stated below and is subject to the special provisions and limitations stated in my Physician Orders for Scope of Treatment (POST) form, a living will, or similar document executed by me, if any. Additional statement of desires, special provisions, and limitations:

```
┌─────────────────────────────────────────────────────────────┐
│                                                             │
│                                                             │
│                                                             │
│                                                             │
│                                                             │
│                                                             │
│                                                             │
│                                                             │
│                                                             │
│                                                             │
│                                                             │
└─────────────────────────────────────────────────────────────┘
```

(You may attach additional pages or documents if you need more space to complete your statement.)

3. INSPECTION AND DISCLOSURE OF INFORMATION RELATING TO MY PHYSICAL OR MENTAL HEALTH

    A.   General Grant of Power and Authority

           Subject to any limitations in this Directive, my agent has the power and authority to do all of the following:

           (1) Request, review and receive any information, verbal or written, regarding my physical or mental health including, but not limited to, medical and hospital records;

           (2) Execute on my behalf any releases or other documents that may be required in order to obtain this information;

           (3) Consent to the disclosure of this information; and

           (4) Consent to the donation of any of my organs for medical purposes.

(If you want to limit the authority of your agent to receive and disclose information relating to your health, you must state the limitations in paragraph 4, "Statement of Desires, Special Provisions, and Limitations", above.)

    B.   HIPAA Release Authority

My agent shall be treated as I would be with respect to my rights regarding the use and disclosure of my individually identifiable health information or other medical records. This release authority applies to any information governed by the Health Insurance Portability and Accountability Act of 1996 (HIPAA), 42

U.S.C. 1320d and 45 CFR 160 through164. I authorize any physician, health care professional, dentist, health plan, hospital, clinic, laboratory, pharmacy, or other covered health care provider, any insurance company, and the Medical Information Bureau, Inc. or other health care clearinghouse that has provided treatment or services to me, or that has paid for or is seeking payment from me for such services, to give, disclose and release to my agent, without restriction, all of my individually identifiable health information and medical records regarding any past, present or future medical or mental health condition, including all information relating to the diagnosis of HIV/AIDS, sexually transmitted diseases, mental illness, and drug or alcohol abuse. The authority given my agent shall supersede any other agreement that I may have made with my health care providers to restrict access to or disclosure of my individually identifiable health information. The authority given my agent has no expiration date and shall expire only in the event that I revoke the authority in writing and deliver it to my health care provider

4. SIGNING DOCUMENTS, WAIVERS, AND RELEASES

Where necessary to implement the health care decisions that my agent is authorized by this Directive to make, my agent has the power and authority to execute on my behalf all of the following:

(a)   Documents titled, or purporting to be, a "Refusal to Permit Treatment" and/or a "Leaving Hospital Against Medical Advice"; and

(b)   Any necessary waiver or release from liability required by a hospital or physician.

5. DESIGNATION OF ALTERNATE AGENTS

(You are not required to designate any alternate agents but you may do so. Any alternate agent you designate will be able to make the same health care decisions as the agent you designated in paragraph 1 above, in the event that agent is unable or ineligible to act as your agent. If an alternate agent you designate is your spouse, he or she becomes ineligible to act as your agent if your marriage is thereafter dissolved.)

If the person designated as my agent in paragraph 1 is not available or becomes ineligible to act as my agent to make a health care decision for me or loses the mental capacity to make health care decisions for me, or if I revoke that person's appointment or authority to act as my agent to make health care decisions for me, then I designate and appoint the following persons to serve as my agent to make health care decisions for me as authorized in this Directive, such persons to serve in the order listed below:

146

A.   First Alternate Agent

      Name: _____

      Address: _____

                        _____

      Telephone Number: _____

B.   Second Alternate Agent

      Name: _____

      Address: _____

                        _____

      Telephone Number: _____

C.   Third Alternate Agent

      Name: _____

      Address: _____

                        _____

      Telephone Number: _____

6. PRIOR DESIGNATIONS REVOKED

I revoke any prior durable power of attorney for healthcare. DATE AND SIGNATURE OF PRINCIPAL

(You must date and sign this Living Will and Durable Power of Attorney for Health Care.)

I sign my name to this Statutory Form Living Will and Durable Power of Attorney for Health Care on the date set forth at the beginning of this Form at:

_____

(Signature)   (City, State)

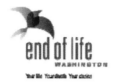

DURABLE POWER OF ATTORNEY FOR HEALTH CARE and HEALTH CARE DIRECTIVE
of:

_____

{Your name here.}

This document states my choices about use of life-sustaining medical treatment and comfort care. It is meant to inform and guide whoever will make health care decisions for me, if I become unable to make my own health care decisions. I understand that such inability may only be temporary. When I can make my own health care decisions I want to do so.

Even when I cannot make my own health care decisions, I want my physician and my health care decision maker(s) to talk to me honestly about my condition and treatment.

I want this directive to remain in effect after my death for autopsy, organ donation, use of my body for medical research, and for my agent to arrange for the disposition of my remains, if I authorize that in section 9.

1. MY HEALTH CARE AGENT

I appoint as my primary agent:

Name _____

Address _____

Telephone _____
              (day)   (evening)   (mobile)

My alternate agent {optional}:

If my primary agent is unable or unwilling to serve, or is unavailable when decisions need to be made for me, then I name this alternate agent:

Name _____

Address _____

Telephone _____
              (day)   (evening)   (mobile)

If my alternate agent acts for me because my primary agent is unavailable, I intend that the alternate agent act only until my primary agent is available.

2. THE AUTHORITY I GIVE MY AGENT

I grant my agent complete authority to make all decisions about my health care. This includes, but is not limited to (a) consenting, refusing consent, and withdrawing consent for medical treatment recommended by my physicians, including life-sustaining treatments; (b) requesting particular medical treatments; (c) employing and dismissing health care providers; (d) changing my health care insurers; (e) signing a Physician Orders for Life-Sustaining Treatment (POLST) form; (f) transferring me to another facility, private home, or other place; and (g) accessing my medical records and information. This authority applies to information governed by the Health Insurance Portability and Accounting Act (HIPAA) of 1996 and any further changes to HIPAA.

3. WHY I AM MAKING THIS DOCUMENT/ HOW TO MAKE HEALTH CARE DECISIONS FOR ME

I want whoever makes health care decisions for me to do as I would want in the circumstances, based on the choices I express in this document. I do not want others to substitute their choices for mine because they disagree with my choices or because they think their choices are in my best interest. I do not want my intentions to be rejected because someone thinks that if I had more information when I completed this document, or if I had known certain medical facts that developed later, I would change my mind. If what I would want is not known, then I want decisions to be made in my best interest, based on (a) my values, (b) the contents of this document, and (c) medical information provided by my health care providers.

_____I have completed and attached an additional statement of my values.
{Optional}

4. WHEN I DO NOT WANT LIFE-SUSTAINING TREATMENT

I value life very much, but I believe that to be kept alive in certain circumstances is worse than death. If I initial an item in this section it means that if such an initialed life-threatening event should occur, I would not want to receive life-sustaining treatment. I want my caregivers to focus on comfort care and pain management, and I should be allowed to die as peacefully as possible: {initial all that apply}

_____ a. Unconsciousness or coma that probably will prevent me from communicating, permanently.

_____ b. Irreversible dementia such as Alzheimer's disease.

_____ c. Total dependence on others for my care because of physical deterioration, which is probably permanent.

_____ d. Pain which probably cannot be eliminated, or can be eliminated only by sedating me so heavily that I cannot converse.

_____ e. Below are other circumstances in which I would not want life-sustaining treatment:
{Optional}

5. WHEN I MAY WANT TEMPORARY USE OF LIFE-SUSTAINING TREATMENT

I understand that I could become unconscious or unable to communicate, *temporarily*. If I were to become unconscious or unable to communicate temporarily, then (initial only *ONE* line):

_____ I would want to receive life-sustaining treatment, for up to weeks (please specify)

_____ I would want to receive life-sustaining treatment for a period of time determined by my health care agent, based on the judgment of my doctor(s).

_____ I still would want no life-sustaining treatment.

6. LIFE-SUSTAINING TREATMENTS I DO NOT WANT

If I experience a condition in which I would not want life-sustaining treatment (as documented in Section 4), or if I experience a quality of life my agent believes I would consider unacceptable, I <u>do not want</u> the following life-sustaining treatments started. If already started, I want them stopped. {Initial all that you **do not** want.}

_____ **All** cardiopulmonary resuscitation (CPR) measures to try to restart my heart and breathing, if those stop, including artificial ventilation, stimulants, diuretics, heart-regulating drugs, or any other treatment for heart failure.

_____ Artificial ventilation when I can no longer breathe on my own.

_____ Heart-regulating drugs, if my heartbeat becomes irregular.

_____ Nutrition and hydration other than ordinary food and water delivered by mouth, if I cannot eat and drink enough to sustain myself.

_____ Surgeries for the purpose of prolonging my life rather than for providing comfort.

_____ Dialysis if my kidneys do not work normally.

_____ Medications, treatments or procedures, when their primary purpose is to prolong life rather than control pain.

_____ Anything else intended to prolong my life.

7. MY WISHES CONCERNING COMFORT CARE AND PAIN MEDICATION

If I am experiencing symptoms such as pain, breathlessness, or visible discomfort, I want treatment to relieve my pain and symptoms and make me comfortable, even if medical providers believe this might unintentionally hasten my death, cause drug dependency, or make me unconscious.

Yes   No

_____   _____

8. IF A HEALTH CARE PROVIDER REFUSES TO HONOR MY DECISIONS OR DECISIONS OF MY HEALTH CARE AGENT

(Cross out this section, if you do not agree.)

If I am ever in a health care facility that refuses to honor my decisions expressed in this document or decisions made for me by my health care agent, I want my agent to take whatever actions he or she decides are appropriate to secure those decisions, including but not limited to changing my physician(s) or moving me out of the facility.

9. MY WISHES CONCERNING OTHER MATTERS

	Yes	No
a. I consent to medical treatments that are experimental.	___	___
b. I want to donate organs/tissues.	___	___
c. I consent to an autopsy.	___	___
d. I consent to use of all or part of my body for medical education or research.	___	___

e. I have named the following individual(s) as my agent(s) for funeral arrangements:

My agent for funeral arrangements:

_____
Name

_____
Address

_____
Telephone (day)   (evening)   (mobile)

My alternate agent for funeral arrangements (if my primary agent is unable or unwilling to serve, or if my agent is a spouse or partner from whom I am separated or divorced when decisions need to be made for me):
{optional}

_____
Name

_____
Address

_____
Telephone (day)   (evening)   (mobile)

f. I want my remains to be disposed of as follows: {describe}

10. IF A COURT APPOINTS A GUARDIAN FOR ME
If I have named a health care agent, I want my agent to be my guardian. If he/she cannot serve, then I want my alternate agent to be my guardian, if I have named an alternate. If the court decides to appoint someone else, I ask that the court require the guardian to consult with my agent (or alternate) concerning all health care decisions that would require my consent if I were acting for myself.

11. HOW THIS DIRECTIVE CAN BE REVOKED OR CANCELED
This directive can be revoked by a written statement to that effect, or by any other expression of intention to revoke. However, if I express disagreement with a particular decision made for me, that disagreement alone is not a revocation of this document. Note: The signed and witnessed Advance Directive with the latest date will take precedence over older Advance Directives.

2. SUMMARY AND SIGNATURE

understand what this document means. If I am ever unable to make my own health care decisions, I am directing whoever makes them for me to do as I have said here. This includes withholding and/or withdrawing life-sustaining medical treatment, which might result in my death occurring sooner than if everything medically possible were done. make this document of my free will, and I believe I have the mental and emotional capacity to do so. I want this ocument to become effective, even if I become incompetent or otherwise disabled.

_____   _____
Signature   Date

Sign only in the presence of two witnesses and a notary, if notarizing.}

3. STATEMENT OF WITNESSES

_____
{Print the legal name of the person making this document on this line.}

is personally known to me, and I believe this person to be of sound mind and to have completed this document voluntarily. I affirm I am at least 18 years old, not related to the signer of this document by blood, marriage, or adoption, and am not their health care agent named in this document. As far as I know I am not a beneficiary of the signer's will or any codicil, and I have no claim against their estate. I am not directly involved in their health care, and I am not an employee of their physician or a health care facility where the person making this document may reside. I am not a home care provider for this person, nor am I a care provider at an adult family home or long-term care facility in which this person resides.

Witness 1   **Witness 2**

_____ _____   _____ _____
Signature   Date   Signature   Date

_____ _____   _____ _____
Printed Name   Phone   Printed Name   Phone

_____   _____
Address   Address

NOTARIZATION {optional}

STATE OF WASHINGTON   County of _____

I certify that I know or have satisfactory evidence that _____ signed this document and acknowledged it to be their free and voluntary act for the uses and purposes mentioned in this document.

Dated this _____ day _____ of 20_____

_____
NOTARY PUBLIC in and for the State of Washington Residing at

_____

My commission expires _____

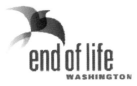

end of life
WASHINGTON
Your life. Your death. Your choice.

LIVING WITH DEMENTIA MENTAL HEALTH ADVANCE DIRECTIVE OF:

_____
(Print your name here.)

As a person with capacity, I willfully and voluntarily execute this mental health advance directive, so that my choices regarding my mental health care and Alzheimer's/dementia care will be carried out in circumstances when I am unable to express my instructions and preferences regarding my future care. If I live in a state that has not adopted laws that provide me with the legal right to make this advance directive, then I want this document to be used as a guide for those who make decisions on my behalf when I am no longer capable of making them for myself.

The fact that I may have left blanks in this directive does not affect its validity in any way. I intend that all completed sections be followed.

I understand that nothing in this directive, including any refusal of treatment that I consent to, authorizes any health care provider, professional person, health care facility, or agent appointed in this directive to use or threaten to use abuse, neglect, financial exploitation, or abandonment to carry out my directive.

I intend this Living With Dementia Mental Health Advance Directive to take precedence over any other mental health directives I have previously executed, to the extent that they are inconsistent with this Living With Dementia Mental Health Advance Directive.

I understand that there are some circumstances where my provider may not have to follow my directive, specifically if compliance would be in violation of the law or accepted standards of care.

1. WHEN AND HOW LONG I WANT THIS DOCUMENT TO APPLY

(Initial only one – a., b., or c. – and draw a line through the others)

a) _____ I intend that this directive become effective **immediately** upon signing and that it remains valid and in effect until revoked according to the terms specified in section 16 or until my death.

b) _____ I intend that this directive become effective if I become incapacitated to the extent that I am unable to make informed consent decisions or provide informed consent for my care, as determined by my treating physician, and that it remain valid and in effect until revoked according to the terms specified in section 16 or until my death.

c) _____ I intend that this directive become effective when any of the following circumstances, symptoms, or behaviors occur, and that it remain valid and in effect until revoked according to the terms specified in section 16 or until my death: *(Initial all that apply, and draw a line through the rest.)*

   1. _____ I am no longer able to communicate verbally.

   2. _____ I can no longer feed myself.

   3. _____ I can no longer recognize my partner/spouse.

   4. _____ I put myself or my family or others in danger because of my actions or behaviors.

   5. Other *(describe)*:

2. WHEN I MAY REVOKE THIS DIRECTIVE

I intend that I be able to revoke this directive: *(Initial one, and draw a line through the other.)*

_____ Only when I have capacity: I understand that choosing this option means I may only revoke this directive if I have capacity. I further understand that if I choose this option and become incapacitated while this directive is in effect, I may receive treatment that I specify in this directive, even if I object at the time.

_____ Even if I am incapacitated: I understand that choosing this option means that I may revoke this directive even if I am incapacitated. I further understand that if I choose this option and revoke this directive while I am incapacitated I may not receive treatment that I specify in this directive, even if I want the treatment.

3. MY MENTAL HEALTH CARE AGENT

I appoint the following person as my primary mental health care agent to make mental health care treatment decisions for me as authorized in this document and request that this person be notified immediately when this directive becomes effective: *(Optional, but highly recommended.)*

Name _____

Address _____

Telephone _____

(day)   (evening)   (mobile)

If the person named above is my partner or spouse at the time I make this document: {Initial one and put a line through the other. If your primary mental health care agent is not your spouse or partner, cross this section out.}

_____ His or her authority to act is hereby revoked if I am separated or divorced from her or him.

_____ His or her authority to act shall be unaffected if I am separated or divorced from her or him.
In the event that my primary mental health care agent is unable, unavailable, or unwilling to serve, or I revoke his or her authority to serve, then I name this alternate mental health care agent and request that this person be notified immediately when this directive becomes effective or when the primary mental health care agent is no longer my agent: *(Optional, but highly recommended.)*

Name _____

Address _____

Telephone _____

(day)   (evening)   (mobile)

If my alternate mental health care agent acts for me because my first agent is unavailable, I intend that the alternate act only while my first agent is unavailable.

4. THE AUTHORITY I GIVE MY MENTAL HEALTH CARE AGENT

I grant my mental health care agent complete authority to make all decisions about mental health care on my behalf. This includes, but is not limited to (a) consenting, refusing consent, and withdrawing consent for mental health treatment recommended by my physicians and other medical providers; (b) requesting particular mental health treatments consistent with any instructions and/or limitations I have set forth in this directive; (c) accessing my medical records and information pertaining to my mental health care; (d) employing and dismissing mental health care providers; and (e) removing me from any mental health care facility to another facility, a private home, or other place. I authorize and request that all "covered entities" under the Health Insurance Portability and Accounting Act of 1996, as hereafter amended, release and disclose full and complete protected medical information to my health care agent named herein. Such information should include, but not be limited to, medical records, office notes, laboratory results, radiology and other visualization records, prescription records, medical opinions, and all other materials that might assist in medical decision-making or a determination of my capacity. I understand that this information may include information about sexually transmitted diseases, AIDS, HIV, and the use/abuse of alcohol and drugs. This consent is subject to revocation at any time except to the extent that the entity which is to make the disclosure has already taken action in reliance on it. If not previously revoked, this authorization will terminate upon my death.

The authority conferred herein shall be exercisable notwithstanding my disability or incapacity.

5. HOW TO MAKE MENTAL HEALTH CARE DECISIONS AND IMPLEMENT THIS DIRECTIVE

I want whoever makes mental health care decisions for me to do as I would want in the circumstances, based on the choices I express in this document. If what I would want is not known, then I want decisions to be made in my best interest, based on my values, the contents of this document, and information provided by my health care providers.

I do not want my mental health care agent or others to substitute their choices for mine because they disagree with my choices or because they think their choices are in my best interests. I do not want my intentions to be rejected because someone thinks that if I had more information when I completed this document, or if I had known certain medical facts that developed later, I would change my mind.

6. PERSONAL HISTORY AND CARE VALUES STATEMENT

(Optional. If you attach a statement, initial this. If not, draw a line through it.)

_____ I have completed and attached an additional statement describing why I am making this metal health advance directive and/or to provide information about the important people in my life, some personal history, general values around care, or anything else that is not addressed by this document.

7. PREFERENCES AND INSTRUCTIONS ABOUT MY CARE AND TREATMENT

a. Preferences regarding care in my home.

(1) **I prefer that my personal care and assistance be provided by:** *(Number the choices below, using the number 1 for your first choice, 2 for your second choice, etc. Draw a line through those that do not apply.)*

_____ Family members who would do so voluntarily.

_____ Individuals who are not family members who would do so voluntarily.

_____ Family members who are hired to provide my care.

_____ Individuals who are not family members who are hired to provide my care.

_____ Other *(describe)*:

(2) **I have the following cultural, religious, and/or gender preferences about my care and assistance:**
(Optional. If you do not have any preferences, draw a line through this space.)

b. Preferences and instructions involving out-of-home placements.

I recognize that I may need to receive care outside of my home – even in my least desirable setting (a nursing home or other placement) – when my care at home becomes too burdensome or difficult to manage. This may be necessary if I become combative, aggressive, incontinent, resistant to care, or too difficult to transfer. If my mental health care agent decides that I need to live in a setting outside of my home, then the following are my preferred locations and settings, in order of preference:

(1) **The location where I would prefer to live:** *(Number the choices below, using the number 1 for your first choice, 2 for your second choice, etc. Draw a line through those that do not apply.)*

_____ With/near the following family member or other loved one near my current home:

_____

_____ With/near the following family member or other loved one far away from my current home:

_____

_____ Near my current home.

_____ Other *(describe)*:

(2) **The setting where I would prefer to live:** *(Number the choices below, using the number 1 for your first choice, 2 for your second choice, etc. Draw a line through those that do not apply.)*

_____ Adult family home. Name: *(optional)*

_____ Assisted living facility. Name: *(optional)*

_____ Nursing home. Name: *(optional)*

_____ Specialized memory care unit. Name: *(optional)*

_____ Moving in with family. Name: *(optional)*

_____ Other *(describe)*:

(3) **If an assessment and/or recommendations about my ability to remain in my home become necessary, the following person/people or agency/agencies is preferred:** *(Optional. If you do not have a preference, draw a line through this space.)*

c. Preferences and instructions about dealing with combative, assaultive, or aggressive behaviors, with authority to consent to inpatient treatment. *(Initial all that apply, and draw a line through those that do not.)*

(1) I recognize that sometimes people with Alzheimer's/dementia become aggressive, assaultive, or combative, despite good care. If this happens, and emergency or other treatment is necessary: *(Initial one or the other directly below; i.e., give your consent or do not consent. If neither is initialed, or you do not consent to voluntary admission to inpatient treatment, commitment could still occur without consideration of the provisions in the "I consent..." statement.)*

_____ I consent and authorize my mental health care agent to consent to voluntary admission to inpatient treatment for up to 14 days, if deemed appropriate by my agent and treating physician. I prefer to receive treatment in a facility specializing in Alzheimer's/dementia care to work on the reduction of my behavioral symptoms and stabilization of my condition.

_____ I do not consent to voluntary admission to inpatient treatment.

(2) _____ I want treatment from trained caregivers who know me and my history, and who know how to handle the situation.

(3) _____ My preference is to be admitted to the specialized geriatric or dementia care unit at

_____

or a similar facility, if available.

(4) _____ My preference is not to be admitted to the following facility or facilities:
(Optional. If you do not have a preference, draw a line through this space.)

d. Preferences regarding the financing of my care.
I know that the cost of my care could become high over the course of my illness. I have the following preferences regarding the financing of my care: *(Initial all that apply. Draw a line through those that do not.)*

_____ My hope is that my care costs will not consume the lifetime of savings I have reserved for retirement and for my children or other heirs at my death.

_____ I want my partner/spouse to maintain the standard of living we now have as much as possible.

_____ I want to preserve as much as possible of my income, assets, and savings for my partner/spouse, children, and heirs. Please use all available planning options to meet this goal, including, but not limited to: *(Cross out any that you do not agree with or that are not applicable.)*

(1) Medicaid planning.
(2) Gifting.
(3) Divorce or legal separation.
(4) Changing estate planning documents.
(5) Tax planning.

_____ Please use my income, assets, and savings to buy the highest quality private care for me.

_____ If my savings run out, I want my home to be sold to finance any further care I need.

_____ I prefer public assistance only if no other option exists for paying for my care.

e. Preferences regarding future intimate relationships.

_1._ Continuation of my intimate relationships with my partner/spouse: *(Initial all that apply. Draw a line through those that do not. Cross out this entire section if it is not applicable.)*

_____ My intimate relationship with my partner/spouse,

*(name here)*_____, is important to both of us.

_____ I consent to maintaining our sexual relationship even in the event that we dissolve our partnership or legal domestic partnership or divorce.

_____ We want to maintain our sexual relationship for as long as possible.

_____ I know that I may forget my partner/spouse as my Alzheimer's/dementia progresses. Even if this happens, I want to continue to be intimate for as long as my partner/spouse wants to and feels comfortable doing so.

_____ If I need nursing home care, I request the privacy needed for us to continue our relationship, as required by law.

_____ I completely trust my partner/spouse to make any judgments about the continuation of our intimate relationship, including when to stop if s/he is no longer comfortable.

_____ Other preference(s):

(2) Preferences regarding my partner/spouse having relationships outside the bounds of our partnership/marriage or other commitment, legally recognized or otherwise: *(Initial all that apply. Draw a line through those that do not. Cross out this entire section if it is not applicable.)*

_____ I understand that my illness may last a long time, and that I likely will no longer recognize or be able to function emotionally or sexually for my partner/spouse. I also care deeply that my partner/spouse not continue to be a victim of this disease and that s/he live her/his life to the fullest. This could include becoming involved in other relationships. I would not consider this a violation of our vows to each other. Rather, I hope that s/he does seek out companionship and intimacy when I can no longer provide that in the relationship.

_____ Our moral, religious, and/or ethical values dictate that we remain faithful to one another through sickness and in health. We have both discussed this, and believe that a relationship outside our partnership/marriage or other committed relationship is not permissible and should not be pursued.

_____ I completely trust my partner/spouse to make any judgments about having relationships outside the bounds of our partnership/marriage, or other committed relationship.

_____ Other preference(s):

(3) Preference regarding future intimate relationships for myself: *(Initial all that apply. Draw a line through those that do not.)*

_____ I know that residents at long-term care facilities sometimes develop relationships with each other that can result in a less depressing and/or happier time for both. I am not completely opposed to my having such a relationship if, in my mental health care agent's judgment, I seem happier and am not coerced in any way.

_____ My moral, religious, and/or ethical beliefs preclude my engagement in any other relationship besides my partnership/marriage, or other committed relationship, whether legal or otherwise. I do not consent to any other intimate relationships, even if I appear to be happier at the time.

_____ Other preference(s):

(4) Preferences regarding my pet(s). *(If you have a pet or pets, write your preferences here. If not, draw a line through this space.)*

8. CONSENT TO PARTICIPATION IN EXPERIMENTAL ALZHEIMER'S/DEMENTIA DRUG TRIALS

(If you initial a, b, or c, or any combination of a, b, or c, you must draw a line through d. If you initial d, you must draw a line through a, b, and c. Draw a line through any that you do not initial.)

a) _____ I consent to participation in any clinical drug trials for drugs that have the potential to ameliorate the symptoms of Alzheimer's/dementia or prevent the full onset of the disease. I not only hope to improve my own health, but also to contribute to research to find a cure for the disease. I give my mental health care agent full power to consent on my behalf to my participation in any such study, considering my preferences regarding side effects.

b) _____ I do not want to take medications that have the following side effects or have the following treatments: {optional}

c) _____ If my memory loss can be slowed down by the experimental drug(s), I am willing to participate in the trial even if it could lead to my earlier death. I would rather die sooner but with my memory more intact.

d) _____ I do not consent to participation in any drug trials.

9. CONSENT REGARDING SUSPENSION OF MY DRIVING PRIVILEGES

(Initial only one, and draw a line through the other.)

_____ My ability to drive is a very important part of my maintenance of independence. I enjoy driving and want to continue to do so as long as I am safe. On the other hand, I know that the time will come when I no longer have the ability to drive safely. I trust my physician(s) or other skilled health care professional(s) who are providing my treatment. *(Name of health care professional(s) here; optional. If you do not want to name someone, put lines through these spaces.)*

_____

If s/he is not available, I want any other skilled health care professional to test my visual and mental acuity to determine if I am no longer safe to drive.

_____ I trust my mental health care agent's judgment on this issue. If my mental health care agent determines that I am unfit to drive, I consent to my driving privileges being suspended. If I continue to drive or attempt to drive after this, I agree to my keys being hidden or taken away from me and/or access to my car being eliminated.

10. REGARDING A HEALTH CARE INSTITUTION REFUSING TO HONOR MY WISHES
(Initial all that reflect your views. Draw a line through any that do not.)

_____ I understand that circumstances beyond my control may cause me to be admitted to a health care or long-term care facility whose policy is to decline to follow advance directives that conflict with certain religious or other beliefs or organizational policies. If I am a patient in such a health care institution or long-term care facility when this Alzheimer's/Dementia Mental Health Advance Directive takes effect, I direct that my consent to admission shall not constitute implied consent to procedures, policies, or courses of treatment mandated by religious or other policies of the institution or facility, if those procedures, policies, or courses of treatment conflict with this mental health advance directive.

_____ If the health care or long-term care facility in which I am a patient declines to follow my wishes as set out in this mental health advance directive, I direct that I be transferred, if possible, in a timely manner to another institution or facility which will agree to honor the instructions set forth in this mental health advance directive.

11. IF A COURT APPOINTS A GUARDIAN FOR ME

If a guardian is appointed by a court to make mental health decisions for me, I intend this document to take precedence over all other means of ascertaining my intent and preferences. The appointment of a guardian of my estate or my person or any other decision-maker shall not give that guardian or decision-maker the power to revoke, suspend, or terminate this Directive or the powers of my mental health care agent, except as authorized by law.

In the event the court appoints a guardian who will make decisions regarding my mental health treatment, I nominate the following person as my guardian:

Name _____

Address _____

Telephone _____
          (day)   (evening)   (mobile)

© Lisa Brodoff & Robb Miller/2012 ■ Commercial distribution prohibited ■ Copying permitted for personal use only ■ 5/19 ■ Page 8
PO Box 61369 Seattle WA 98141 ■ 206.256.1636 ■ info@EndofLifeWA.org ■ EndofLifeWA.org

12. OTHER DOCUMENTS

In planning for my health care, estate, and potential incapacity, I have executed the following documents: *(Initial and provide information for all that apply. Draw a line through those that do not.)*

_____ **General Power of Attorney:** *(Name and contact info of primary agent.)*

Name _____
Address _____
Telephone _____
           (day)   (evening)   (mobile)

_____ **Durable Power of Attorney for Finances:** *(Name and contact info of primary agent.)*

Name _____
Address _____
Telephone _____
           (day)   (evening)   (mobile)

_____ **Durable Power of Attorney for Health Care:** *(Name and contact info of primary health care agent.)*

Name _____
Address _____
Telephone _____
           (day)   (evening)   (mobile)

_____ **Living Will/Health Care Directive/Directive to Physicians:** *(Name and contact info of person who has a copy.)*

Name _____
Address _____
Telephone _____
           (day)   (evening)   (mobile)

_____ **Physician Orders for Life-Sustaining Treatment (POLST):**
(Optional; name and contact information of person who has access to your POLST.)

Name _____
Address _____
Telephone _____
           (day)   (evening)   (mobile)

_____ **Other Document:** *(Optional; name here:.)*

Name _____
Address _____
Telephone _____
           (day)   (evening)   (mobile)

3. SUMMARY AND SIGNATURE

I understand what this document means. I make this document of my free will, and I believe I have the mental and emotional capacity to do so.

By signing here, I indicate that I understand the purpose and effect of this document, and that I am giving my informed consent to the treatments and/or admission that I have consented to, or that I have authorized my agent to consent to, in this directive. I intend that my consent in this directive be construed as being consistent with the elements of informed consent under RCW Chapter 7.70 in the State of Washington or applicable law in other states.

Signature of person making this document _____.

Date_____

(Sign only in the presence of two witnesses and a notary, if notarizing.)

4. STATEMENT OF WITNESSES

This directive was signed and declared by

(Print your name – not the names of your witnesses – on the following line.)

_____ to be her/his directive. It was signed in
our presence at her/his request. We declare that at the time of the creation of this directive

(Print your name – not the names of your witnesses – on the following line.)

_____ is personally known to us and, according to our best
knowledge and belief, has capacity at this time and does not appear to be acting under duress, undue influence, or fraud. We further declare that none of us is:

a. A person designated to make medical decisions on the principal's behalf.

b. A health care provider or professional person directly involved with the provision of care to the principal at the time the directive is executed.

c. An owner, operator, employee, or relative of an owner or operator of a health care facility or long-term care facility in which the principal is a patient or resident.

d. A person who is related by blood, marriage, legal domestic partnership, or adoption to the person, or with whom the person making this document has a dating relationship as defined in RCW 26.50.010 in the State of Washington or applicable law in other states.

e. An incapacitated person.

f. A person who would benefit financially if the principal undergoes mental health treatment.

g. A minor.

WITNESS 1		WITNESS 2	
_____	_____	_____	_____
Signature	Date	Signature	Date
_____	_____	_____	_____
Printed Name	Phone	Printed Name	Phone
_____		_____	
Address		Address	

NOTARIZATION *(optional)*

STATE OF COUNTY OF

I certify that I know or have satisfactory evidence that signed this document and acknowledged it to be his/her free and voluntary act for the uses and purposes mentioned in this document.

_____

NOTARY PUBLIC in and for the State of

_____

Residing at

_____

My commission expires

_____

15. RECORD OF DIRECTIVE

I have given a copy of this directive to the following persons:

_____
_____
_____
_____

6. REVOCATION OF MY LIVING WITH DEMENTIA MENTAL HEALTH ADVANCE DIRECTIVE

(Initial either 1 or 2, and draw a line through the one you did not initial. If you initial 1, then list the sections that you are revoking by number. For example: "Sections 2, 6, and 7.")

_____ 1. I am revoking the following part(s) of this directive (specify):

_____

_____

_____

_____

_____ 2. I am revoking this entire directive.

By signing here, I indicate that I understand the purpose and effect of my revocation and that no person is bound by any revoked provision(s). I intend this revocation to be interpreted as if I had never completed the revoked provision(s).

_____   _____

Signature of person who made this document   Date

ADVANCE DIRECTIVE (STATE OF VIRGINIA)
with Sections for Medical, Mental, and End-of-Life Health Care

I,_____(date of birth
_____),make this advance directive in case I am not able to make health care decisions for myself. This advance directive says what I do want and what I do not want for my health care.

Section 1: Health Care Decision Maker (My "Agent")

A. Who I Pick to be My Agent

I appoint_____to make health caredecisions for me when I cannot make those decisions myself.

First agent's contact information:

Ph. No. (home):_____(cell):

_____Ph. No. (work):

_____Email:

_____Home   Address:

_____

_____

I also pick a person to be my agent if the first person I picked is not available, able orwilling to act as my agent. My back-up agent is:

_____

Back-up agent's contact information:

Ph. No. (home):_____(cell):

Ph. No. (work):_____Email:

_____Home   Address:

_____

My agent will have full power to make health care decisions for me based on this advance directive. My agent will have this power only during a time when I am notable to make informed decisions about my health care.

I want my agent to follow what I have written in this advance directive. My agent mayalso be guided by information that I have given my agent in other ways, such as in conversation. If my agent cannot tell what choice I would have made, then my agent should choose what he or she believes to be in my best interests.

I want my agent and health care providers to communicate with me and consider myviews even when I am unable to make my own decisions and the agent has the power to make decisions for me.

165

B. What My Agent Can Do On My Behalf

If you appointed an agent on page 1, these are the powers that he/she will have.

You may cross through any powers that you do not want to give your agent.

If you have questions about what the powers mean, you might find the "What it means to give powers to your health care agent" sheet helpful. It can be found on the www.VirginiaAdvance Directives.org website.

Power 5 Option:

Virginia law lets you authorize your agent to make the decision about admission to a mental health care facility on the basis of just one professional examining you and determining you cannot make an informed decision. Any other treatment decisions beyond admission to a mental health care facility will still require the usual determination process by

(a) your attending physician + (b) a second physician or clinical psychologist. If you want to include this part of Power 5, you need to check the box.

Power 9: If you have any specific instructions about visitation, you need to say so on page 8. Note: other laws and regulations may limit an agent's power to make visitation decisions.

You may add any additional details about the powers (e.g., "My agent may not fire Dr. Smith").

My agent will have power…

1. To consent to or refuse consent to or withdraw consent to any type of health care, treatment, surgical procedure, diagnostic procedure, and medication.

> This may include use of a breathing machine, tube feeding, IV fluids, or CPR. It also includes higher than recommended doses of pain-relieving medication in order to relieve pain. This applies even if the medication carries the risk of addiction or of unintentionally hurrying my death.

2. To ask for, receive and review oral or written information about the health care decisions that need to be made. This includes medical and hospital records. My agent can also allow this information to be shared with providers as needed to carry out my advance directive wishes.

3. To hire and fire my health care providers.

4. To consent to my admission to, transfer to, or discharge from a hospital, hospice, nursing home, assisted living facility or other health care facility.

5. To consent to my admission to a mental health care facility when it is recommended by my health care providers.

> The admission can be for up to the maximum time permitted by current law. At the time I made this advance directive the maximum was ten (10) calendar days.

> ☐ Power 5 option: My agent may exercise this power after one of the following professionals determines that I am not able to make an informed decision about admission: an attending physician, a psychiatrist or clinical psychologist, a psychiatric nurse practitioner, a clinical social worker, or a designee of the local community services board who is trained and certified to assess capacity.

6. To continue to act as my agent as long as I am unable to decide for myself, even if I state that I want to fire my agent.

7. To consent to my participation in any health care study if the study offers the chance of therapeutic benefit to me.

> The study must be approved by an institutional review board or research review committee according to applicable federal or state law.

8. To consent to my participation in any health care study that aims to increase scientific understanding of a condition that I may have or to promote human well-being, even though it offers no direct benefit to me.

> The study must be approved by an institutional review board or research review committee according to applicable federal or state law.

9. To make decisions about visitation when I am admitted to any health care facility. My agent must follow any directions on visitation I give on page 8 of this advance directive.

10. To take any lawful actions needed to carry out these decisions. This may include signing releases of liability to medical providers or other health care forms.

Additional details:

Part C lets you give your agent the power to consent to treatment that you say "no" to. This power applies only if you cannot make informed decisions.

If you <u>do not</u> want to give your agent this power, you can skip or cross through Part C.

This power has two parts:

1. You can give your agent the power to act over your objection <u>to inpatient mentalhealth admission</u> *and/or*

2. You can give your agent the power to act over your objection <u>to other health care</u>

You can also exclude specific treatments that you always want to be able to object to.

IMPORTANT: You need to have one of the following licensed professionals sign this page to make Part C legally binding: a physician, clinical psychologist, physician assistant, nurse practitioner, professional counselor, or clinical social worker. This professional checks that you understand the consequences of giving your agent the powers described on this page.

If you are not completing Part C, you do not need to have this page signed.

C. What My Agent Can Do Over My Objection

When I am not able to make informed decisions about my health care, I may say "no" to treatment that I actually need. If my agent and my physician believe I need that treatment, my agent has the power:

☐ _____ 1. To consent to my admission to a mental health care facility aspermitted by law, even if I object.

and/or

☐ _____ 2. To consent to other health care that is permitted by law, even if Iobject.

This authority includes all health care except for what I have written in thenext sentence or elsewhere in this document.

My agent does **not** have the authority to consent to _____

_____ over my objection.

I am a licensed: ☐ physician, ☐ clinical psychologist, ☐ physician assistant, ☐ nurse practitioner, ☐ professional counselor, ☐ clinical social worker. I am familiar with the person who has made this advance directive for health care. I attest that this person is presently capable of making an informed decision andthat this person understands the consequences of the special powers given to his/her agent by this Subsection C of this advance directive.

_____

Signature   Date

_____

Printed Name and Address

167

You may use **Section 2** to give directions about your health care. You may skip over or cross out any parts that you do not want to fill out. You can use these partseven if you do not pick an agent.

Section 2: My Health Care Preferences and Instructions

My preferences and instructions for my health care are written in this section. My health care agent and any health care providers working with me are directed to provide care in line with my stated instructions and preferences. *I understand that myproviders do not have to follow preferences or instructions that are medically or ethically inappropriate or against the law.*

A. My Health Conditions and Current Treatments

Part A lets you provide background information to your health care providers. Itincludes no instructions.

1. My current health condition(s) and important things about my condition(s)that health care providers should know:

2. Symptom(s) that indicate I need prompt medical attention:

If you have symptoms that show you need mental healthcare, you can write them hereand on page 6.

3. My medications and dosages as of_____ / ____/20____ :

Medication	Dose	How/when I take it

ỳ See back of this page for more	ỳ See attached list for more

You can also provide medication information by attaching a list of your medications to this AD, or writing where people can get your medication information (e.g., calling your primary care doctor).

4. Other important information regarding medications (allergies, side effects):

B. Information Sharing

My current providers, who have information to help with my care, are:

Name	Provider type (e.g., PCP, psychiatrist)	Phone number

168

C. Emergency Contacts

I authorize the health care providers and other people helping me to contact my health care agent. This authorization includes if I am admitted to a mental healthfacility.

I also authorize them to contact the following people to share information about mylocation, condition and needs:

Name:_____ Relationship to me: _____

Ph. No. (home):_____(cell):_____

Ph. No. (work):_____Email:_____

Home Address:_____

Limit of details to share, if any: _____

Name: _____Relationship to me: _____

Ph. No. (home):_____(cell):_____

Ph. No. (work):_____Email:_____

Home Address:_____

Limit of details to share, if any: _____

D. Medication

1. Medication Preferences

Part D lets you give your preferences for medications.You may refer to specific medications or types of medications.

Your physician must consideryour preferences. But medication decisions must bebased on his or her clinical judgment too.

Your physician is not requiredto follow preferences that are medically or ethically inappropriate.

You have the option of tellingproviders more information about your choices—it can help them to better follow your wishes.

I prefer that the following medications (or classes or types of medication) be tried firstin a crisis or emergency:

Medication name or class	As treatment for...

I prefer these medications because:

169

2. Medication Authorization and Refusal Instructions

<u>General authorization to consent to medications</u>: Generally, I authorize my agent to consent to medications that my treating physician says are appropriate.

<u>Medication refusal instructions</u>: Although I generally authorize my agent to consent to medications, I specifically do **not** consent to the medications listed below. (This includes brand-name, trade-name, or generic equivalents.)

Although I do not consent to these medications, I realize that my condition and needs may change. So, I also state whether my agent can consent to the medication if necessary. My agent should consent only if my physician finds that the medication is clearly the most appropriate treatment for me under the circumstances.

Medication name or class that I do not want	As treatment for...	My agent can authorize it if necessary	
		Yes	No
		Yes	No
		Yes	No

I do not want these medications because:

3. Additional preferences about medications:

E. Mental Health Crisis Intervention

1. My Past Experience

a. Symptoms I might experience during a period of crisis:

b. Interventions that may help me:

In general, your agent cannot authorize and your physician cannot order use of the medications that you refuse here. There are some narrow exceptions permitted by law, such as emergencies.

You may leave the option open for your agent to consent to a refused medication if circumstances indicate the medication really is the most appropriate one under the circumstances.

You have the option of telling providers more information about your choices—it can help them to better follow your instructions.

You can add any other preferences about medication here, such as whether you prefer shots, pills, or liquid forms of medicines.

If you have, previously had, or are at risk of a mental health condition, **Part E** allows you to provide information about your condition and your preferences to help your agent and health care providers meet your needs in a mental health crisis.

Your health care providers must consider your preferences relating to the location and type of care but their ability to follow them may be limited by clinical, legal and administrative requirements.

c. Interventions or other factors that may make things worse:

2. Crisis units, inpatient facilities, and hospitals:

a. I prefer to be treated at the following facilities if 24-hour care is required:

because:

Your health care providers
must consider your
preferences relating to the
location of care but their
ability to follow them may be
limited by clinical, legal and
administrative requirements.

b. I prefer not to be treated at the following facilities:

because:

c. Facility staff can help me by doing the following:

d. I prefer to be transported by:

3. Behavioral emergency interventions: If I am in immediate danger of harming myself or other people, emergency interventions may be medically necessary. I am listing the four types of emergency interventions in order of my preference here.

_____Medication in pill or liquid form

_____Physical restraint

_____Medication by injection

_____Seclusion

I have put them in this order because:

You may use this space to provide any other informationthat is important to your care that may not be addressed above. If you need more space, you may attach additional documents. If youuse attachments, you shouldbe sure to describe them clearly here.

If you gave your agent the power to make visitation decisions, your agent must make visitation decisions based on any instructions you write here.

More information about ECT is available from groups like **NAMI** (*https://www.nami.org/ Learn-More/Treatment*) **and** the Mayo Clinic (*http://www.mayoclinic.org/te sts-procedures*).

You can use **Part G** to request that some tasks be taken care of while you are hospitalized.

Although expressing your wishes could be very useful, these statements do not necessarily have any legal effect. For example, your health care agent is not legally required to pay your bills.

F. Other Health Care Details

1. In General

2. Visitation Instructions

If I am in a health care facility, this is how I want visitation to be handled:

3. Electroconvulsive Therapy (ECT) Instructions

☐ _____A. I authorize my agent to consent to electroconvulsive therapy if mydoctor(s) say that it is medically appropriate.

OR

☐ _____B. I do not consent to electroconvulsive therapy.

G. Life Management Requests

☐ I have a crisis plan that can be found:_____

1. If I am hospitalized, I would like for the following tasks to be carried out <u>at myhome</u>:

2. If I am hospitalized, I would like the following tasks to be carried out in regard to <u>my job and other outside activities and responsibilities</u>:

3. If I am unable to care for my child(ren), then my first choice to care for them is: Name_____

___Relationship:_____ Address:_____

___ Email: _____ Phone (home):___(cell):_____

___ (work): _____

172

H. Life-Prolonging Treatment

1. If my doctor determines that my death is imminent (very close) and medicaltreatment will not help me recover, then:

☐ _____ I do not want any treatments to prolong my life. This includes tube feeding,IV fluids, cardiopulmonary resuscitation (CPR), ventilator/respirator (breathing machine), kidney dialysis or antibiotics. I understand that I still will receive treatment to relieve pain and make me comfortable.

☐ _____ I want all treatments to prolong my life as long as possible within the limitsof generally accepted health care standards. I understand that I will receive treatment to relieve pain and make me comfortable.

☐ _____ Other choices, as follows:

2. If my condition makes me unaware of myself or my surroundings or unable tointeract with others, and it is reasonably certain that I will never recover this awareness or ability even with medical treatment, then:

☐ _____ I do not want any treatments to prolong my life. This includes tube feeding,IV fluids, cardiopulmonary resuscitation (CPR), ventilator/respirator (breathing machine), kidney dialysis or antibiotics. I understand that I still will receive treatment to relieve pain and make me comfortable.

☐ _____ I want all treatments to prolong my life as long as possible within the limitsof generally accepted health care standards. I understand that I will receive treatment to relieve pain and make me comfortable.

☐ _____ I want to try treatments for a period of time in the hope of some improvement of my condition. I suggest _____
as the period of time after which such treatment should be stopped if my condition has not improved. Any agent or surrogate may specify the exact time period in consultation with my physician. I understand that I still will receive treatment to relieve pain and make me comfortable.

☐ _____ Other choices, as follows:

173

If you leave this section blank, your agent will have the authority to donate your organs, eyes and tissues or your whole body. If you do not want your agent to have that authority, write in the box"I do not want to be an organ donor."

If you want to be an organ donor, check only 1 box and initial the line.

If you want to be an organ donor, you may also use this space to write any specific instructions you wish to give about organ donation.

You can also register or change your directions on the donor registry, *www.*

DonateLifeVirginia.org.

Two adult witnesses are needed to make your advance directive valid. Any person over the age of 18 may be a witness. This includes a spouse or relative, as well as employees of health care facilities and physician's offices who act in good faith.

This form meets the requirements of Virginia's Health Care Decisions Act. If you have legal questions about this form or would like to develop a different form tomeet your particular needs, you should talk with an attorney.

Note: If you have added pages with instructions, those pages should be signed and witnessed, too.

This advance directive should be accepted in other states based on "reciprocity" laws that honor valid out of state documents. Check with your health care provider.

Section 3: Organ

☐ _____ I donate my organs, eyes and tissues for use in transplantation, therapy, research and education. I direct that all necessary measures be taken to ensure themedical suitability of my organs, eyes or tissues for donation.

OR

☐ _____ I donate my whole body for research and education.

Section 4: Required Signatures

Right to Revoke: I understand that I may cancel all or part of my AD at any time thatI am able to understand the consequences of doing so.

Affirmation: I am signing below to show that I understand this document and that Imade it voluntarily.

_____   _____
Date   Signature

The above person signed this advance directive in my presence.

_____   _____
Witness Signature   Witness Printed

_____   _____
Witness Signature   Witness Printed

It is your responsibility to provide a copy of your advance directive to your healthcare providers. You also should provide copies to your agent, close relatives and/or friends.

In addition to sharing hard copies, you are encouraged to store your advancedirective in Virginia's free Advance Directive Registry located at the Virginia Department of Health website: https://*www.connectvirginia.org/adr/*. If you have stored your advance directive in the Registry, initial here: _____

INDEX

Page numbers followed by an *f* indicate a figure.

Made in the USA
Columbia, SC
18 November 2021

49016039R00095